The Unfolded Organon

Organon

A Précis of Hahnemann's Sixth Edition

by Peter Crockett

GW00579020

Published by the Homeopathy Allergy Store
15 Westbourne Road
Islington, London N7 8AN
44 (0)20 7700 4234

Printed by
WCS Digital Print
44 (0)20 7278 0950

Typography & Design
Gabrielle Markus

ISBN 0 9519893 2 4

CONTENTS

INTRODUCTION

The Organon is not easy to reference. Even with a good index one has to know the book well to find sought after statements buried in 291 paragraphs and 170 footnotes. Yet it is organised into coherent ideas flowing into one another; I have therefore headed each section and made a table of contents.

In the index I have used a device from Nash's 'Leaders in Homœopathic Therapeutics' of additionally indexing and emboldening the main heading references.

In German, nouns have gender: masculine, feminine, and neuter. This makes it possible to describe complex ideas involving many elements (nouns) in one long paragraph, referring back to each noun by its gendered pronoun 'it'. This works in German with rare confusions when written well. The problem arises when translating into a language which does not have gendered pronouns – e.g., English. Long rambling sentences appear, with clauses that could refer to one of several nouns. It becomes very difficult to hold onto the point, and this is compounded by Hahnemann's style being both complex and pedantic, even in the original German.

I have therefore reduced each paragraph to its fundamental statement, trying to keep the sense while discarding frequent accusatory statements and sometimes unnecessary repetition. This is done with one aim:- to make the Organon clearer. In the same spirit I have left out some long examples of phenomena which add little to meaning; they are all referenced.

There is an idea that the Organon is dense and difficult and not that relevant to contemporary homœopathy. But as one becomes more familiar with the book one begins to realise it's clarity and completeness. The ideas are clear, the language is not. We find information not only on philosophy, but also practical advice on all aspects of long and short term treatment, repeating remedies, chronic disease classifications and how to treat them, how to prepare medicines, provings, and so on. In fact, most of the questions one is ever going to ask of homoeopathy are answered in The Organon of Medicine.

Peter Crockett
8th April 1995,
Islington, London

O mickle is the powerful grace that lies
In herbs, plants, stones, and their true qualities.
                                    Romeo and Juliet II, 3

Section 1

HOMŒOPATHIC MEDICINE

The Physician and His Job

1. The physician's highest and *only* calling is to restore health to the sick, this is called Healing.[1]

> F/N 1: Not to construct hypotheses on the nature of vital processes or give explanations on the phenomena and causes of disease, wrapped in unintelligible words, while sick humanity sighs for aid. We should act and not theorise.

2. The highest aim of healing is to restore health gently and permanently, according to comprehensible principles, in the shortest and safest manner.

3. If we know what is to be cured in disease – the medicinal powers – how to select the remedy – the remedy's correct dose – and the obstacles to cure – then we are *true physicians*.

4. And likewise, if we preserve health – know what disturbs health – and how to remove it.

5. It assists the cure to discover the diseases' *fundamental cause* (which is generally due to a chronic miasm) by knowing the probable *exciting cause* of acute diseases, and the significant points in the history of chronic disease. In your consultation, consider the physical constitution (especially in chronic diseases), moral and intellectual character, occupation, mode of living and habits, social and domestic relations, age, sex life, etc., of the patient.

The Totality of Symptoms

6. The unprejudiced observer only notes the change in health to the body and mind in a disease *(morbid phenomena, accidents, symptoms)* which can be perceived externally by means of his senses, and as felt by the patient and seen by those around him. This represents the disease in its entirety.[2]

> F/N 2: Treat according to the patient's symptoms, not according to preconceived ideas and medicines. We do not need to look for invisible causes. Cure only the observable symptoms.

7. If there is no obvious exciting or maintaining cause[3] that needs removing *(causa occasionalis)* in the patient's general circumstances (or miasm § 5), then the removal of the totality[4] of the symptoms will cure the patient.

> F/N 3: Remove foreign bodies from the eye, loosen tight bandages etc. (There follow a number of examples.)

> F/N 4: Don't treat *single* symptoms. One symptom, like a foot, is not the whole man.

8. After the symptoms have gone the patient is healthy.[5]

> F/N 5: The disease does not remain as *a material something* lurking in some corner of the body once the symptoms have gone.

The Dynamis or Vital Force

9. In health the dynamis or spiritual vital force is the controller of the organism and provides a home for the mind to pursue the higher purpose of our existence.

10. If there is no dynamis or vital force there is no life. The material organism derives all sensation and function[6] from this animating immaterial being.

> F/N 6: Once dead the organism decays, being now subject to the laws of the physical world.

11. When a person falls ill the dynamis or vital force is primarily deranged by the dynamic morbific agent. It expresses itself through *disease symptoms* in the organism.[7]

> F/N 7: An argument based on the idea that unseen forces like magnetism are dynamic hidden energies in the same way as morbid influences. Therefore diseases can be transmitted from a distance without any material connection. Medicines are only medicines in so far as they are able to affect the well being of man through dynamic influence and each will do so in its own characteristic manner. More healing energy is transmitted through minute doses of a medicine than through large material doses. He finishes by asking what raises our arm? A lever, or a conceptual dynamic energy of will?

12. It is the morbidly affected vital force that produces diseases[8] and the morbid derangement or symptoms that reveal the disease. The disappearance of the morbid derangements or symptoms restores the integrity of the vital force and therefore the health of the organism.

> F/N 8: *How* the vital force causes the organism to display symptoms is of no practical use. We only need to know what has been revealed to our senses – the symptoms.

Disease

13. Therefore disease (that does not require surgery) is not separate from the living whole or organism and its animating vital force.

14. All diseases manifest symptoms to the observer.

The Affected Dynamis

15. The affection of the dynamis and the symptoms produced are one. The material organism and dynamis are a unity. Thought separates them to facilitate comprehension.

16. Injurious influences affect the vital force, as a spirit-like dynamis, dynamically. They can only be removed by dynamic[9] medicines, so health can only be restored dynamically.

> F/N 9: Most severe disease can be produced by sufficient disturbance of the vital force through the imagination and also cured by the same means.

17. As cure eliminates all perceptible signs of disease, and removes the inner alteration of the vital force,[10] it follows that the totality of symptoms must be removed in order to remove our inner untunement.[11] Then health is restored.

> F/N 10: A prediction of death can lead to worsening of symptoms and even death itself. This is only possible by the production of an inward change corresponding to the external state. Likewise one can banish signs announcing early death and restore health by suggestion. This can only be possible by the removal of outer as well as inner morbid disturbances.

> F/N 11: God allows us to heal by showing us what we need to remove for cure. His motives would be questionable if he had shrouded them in mystery.

Remedies or Medicines

18. The totality of symptoms, and circumstances observed in each individual case, must be the *sole indication* in choosing a remedy.

19. Medicines only cure if they have the power to alter how a person senses and functions.

20. It is only possible to see the spirit-like power of a medicine through its actions on the state of health – not through an effort of reason.

21. The curative principle in medicines is not perceptible, but we can see that they change the state of health. Remedies can only cure because they bring into play characteristic or peculiar changes in the *healthy individual*. This is how they reveal their curative powers showing each medicine's disease-producing power at the same time as its disease-curing power.

22. To restore health, symptoms must be removed. Medicines become remedies and destroy disease only by their ability to stimulate certain symptoms, creating artificial disease conditions which can eliminate the existing symptoms or natural disease. For this to happen one must look for a medicine which produces a totality of the most similar or opposite symptoms to a disease. (Experience shall prove whether this is done most readily by *similar* or *opposite* medicinal symptoms.[12])

> F/N 12: A third method (to similars or opposites) is the *allopathic* which prescribes medicines that have no direct pathological relation to the morbid state, neither similar nor opposite. The pretext is that we must imitate the instinctive efforts of the dynamis to cure itself. The vital force was made to sustain harmony – not to heal itself. If it did we would never become ill. In disease it expresses untunement through disturbance of normal function and pain. To imitate this is not sensible.

Homœopathic Medicines

23. Persistent symptoms are not destroyed by *opposite* medicines (as in the *antipathic, enantiopathic or palliative* method). They return after improving for a time with increased intensity. (See §§ 58-62 and 69)

24. So only homœopathy is effective because it chooses the remedy most similar to the totality of a case; one that has been tested on the healthy and found to produce an artificial state most similar to the disease in question.

25. Experience[13] teaches us that the medicine that will cure permanently, destroying the symptoms, is the one producing the greatest number of symptoms *similar* to the disease.

> F/N 13: A comment on the questionable practices of some 18th and 19th century approaches to medicine. "Much theory and little investigation."

26. This depends upon the following natural law of homœopathy: *a weaker dynamic affection is permanently extinguished by a stronger one which, though differing in kind, is similar to it in its manifestations.*[14]

> F/N 14: Thus physical and moral maladies are cured. (There follow numerous examples of like curing or overtaking like in the world around us.)

27. Curative medicines therefore must be similar to and stronger (§§ 12-26) than the disease.

28. The premise in paragraphs 25, 26, & 27 is proven by pure experiment and observation in the world. *How it takes place* is unimportant although the following may go some way to explaining.

29. The untuned dynamis is taken over by a stronger and similar artificial disease, *i.e*, the well chosen remedy. Therefore the weaker dynamic disease is extinguished. The dynamis is only concerned with the new artificial disease which gradually wanes leaving the patient cured. The dynamis frees itself more easily from artificial medicinal diseases than natural ones because medicinal diseases have a short action. Natural disease, though weaker, has a longer life, as long as life itself. This applies to every disease that is not entirely surgical, and is based upon the following propositions.

The Effect of Medicines

30. It appears that suitable medicines[15] (partly because we can regulate the dose) alter the organism more than natural disease agents because they can cure them.

> F/N 15: Even though it is stronger than a natural disease the short duration of the action of a medicine (an unnatural disease) means that it can be easily overcome by the vital force .

31. Morbific disease agents do not derange health unconditionally.[16] We fall ill only when our organism is susceptible. They do not produce disease in everyone or at all times.

> F/N 16: Diseases are *not* mechanical or chemical alterations of the material substance of the body and are not dependent upon a material morbific substance. They are spirit-like, conceptual, dynamic derangements of life.

32. Real medicines can at *all* times affect *every* person, natural disease does not do this.

33. People are therefore *unconditionally* susceptible to medicinal forces. Natural diseases affect people *conditionally*.[17]

F/N 17: All children who escaped an epidemic of Scarlatina one year caught it the next. *All* the children who took Belladonna in another epidemic escaped the disease. If medicines can protect from an epidemic they must have a superior capability of affecting our vital force.

34. The greater strength of the artificial disease (or remedy) is not the only reason for cure, it also has to be *as similar as possible* so as to extinguish the disease. Neither dissimilar drugs nor dissimilar diseases can cure the derangement caused by a natural disease.

Dissimilar Diseases

35. To illustrate, let us consider in three different cases what happens when two dissimilar diseases meet in the same person, either due to natural diseases or the use of unsuitable allopathic drugs. We shall prove that neither nature, nor unhomœopathic medicines can cure with a dissimilar stronger disease.

36. 1) If two *dissimilar* diseases in a patient are equally strong or if the *older is stronger,* the older will repel the new disease in both cases. (Examples follow).[18]

F/N 18: A reference to one of the examples quoted.

37. Thus old chronic diseases remain uncured by *allopathic* treatment, even when the treatment is mild,[19] using remedies that do not produce a similar condition to the disease.

F/N 19: But if treated with violent allopathic remedies, other diseases are created in their place which are more dangerous and difficult to treat.

38. 2) If *the second dissimilar disease is stronger* it temporarily suspends and suppresses the first until it runs its course or is cured. Then the

old affection re-appears uncured. This is the case unless they complicate each other which rarely happens in acute diseases. *They never cure each other.* (Examples follow).[20-30]

F/N 20-30: A number of references to the examples quoted.

39. Have physicians not noticed that *dissimilar* drug treatments merely *suspend* disease and do not cure it? (Examples follow).[31]

F/N 31: A reference to an example.

40. 3) *The new disease* after acting for a long time can *join the old dissimilar one* forming a *complex* disease. Each occupies particular regions of the organism characteristically belonging to it. Therefore a syphilitic patient can become psoric and *vice versa.*[32] *Being dissimilar they cannot cure one another.* The venereal symptoms may diminish and be suspended while the psoric eruptions appear but finally the two join together making the patient more diseased and more difficult to cure. In rare instances two dissimilar acute diseases have appeared simultaneously in the same body. (Examples follow).[33-37]

F/N 32: Complex diseases are not an amalgamation but are two dissimilar diseases existing side by side. Cure can be effected by judicious alternation of the best mercurial preparation with the specific psoric remedies in most suitable dose and form.

F/N 33-37: References to various papers illustrating the examples quoted.

41. Two diseases forming a complex disease are much less common than the morbid complications caused by the prolonged use of unsuitable medicines. The medicinal disease gradually combines with the dissimilar chronic trouble. Similarly syphilis with psora or gonorrhœa forms a monstrously complicated disease when treated with unsuitable mercurial preparations.[38]

> F/N 38: For Mercury, besides its homœopathic similarity, has effects unlike those of syphilis (for instance, ulcerations and swelling of the bones) which, when used in large doses, cause new maladies; especially when complicated with psora.

42. Two (or even three) simultaneous diseases can only occur in the same body when they are *dissimilar.* They do not cure or remove one another but remain separate in the organism in their appropriate parts and systems. Because of their lack of similarity they can remain without disparagement to the unity of life.

Similar Diseases

43. The result is totally different when two *similar* diseases meet in an organism – when a similar stronger disease is added to an existing disease. A cure is effected by nature which shows us how to cure.

44. Two *similar* diseases cannot 1) *repel* each other (§§ 36 & 37), 2) *suspend* each other (so the old returns after the new has run its course) (§§ 38 & 39), or 3) *exist next to each other* in the same organism or form a *double* complex disease (§§ 40 & 41).

45. The stronger disease destroys the weaker because of its predominance over the *same* parts of the organism formerly affected by the weaker disease.[39]

> F/N 39: Just as the lamp's flame is extinguished by the stronger sunbeam.

46. Various examples of homœopathic cures brought about by similar natural diseases in nature.[40-57]

> F/N 40-57: References to the above.

47. The above examples teach us what kind of medicine we should choose in order to cure in a way that conforms with natural processes.

48. All the previous examples show dissimilar disease agents do not cure. Only *similar, stronger* ones do.

49. There would be more examples if 1) observers had noted them, and 2) nature was richer in homœopathic diseases.

50. Nature has few homœopathic diseases (besides the miasmatic diseases of constant character like the itch, smallpox[58] and measles) and they[59] are worse than the diseases they cure. Therefore their use would be dangerous and they would need to, in turn, be cured. Also a natural disease 'dose' cannot be reduced. However we can point to many such lucky homœopathic cures by these diseases due to *cure by symptom similarity.*

> F/N 58: And the exanthematous contagious principle present in the cow-pox lymph.

> F/N 59: Namely smallpox and measles.

51. We therefore have an advantage over the choices of nature as there are thousands of curative agents. We can then dilute, subdivide and potentise almost infinitely, reducing the dosage until they are only slightly stronger than the disease they treat. There is no need to attack the organism with violence.

Homœopathy and Allopathy

52. There are only two principle therapies: homœopathic, based on the above observations, and allopathic (heteropathic). They oppose one another and cannot be united. Only someone who does not know either is foolish enough to treat one moment homœopathic and the next allopathic to please the patient.

53. Gentle cures are exclusively homœopathic. This method, seen through the conclusions above (§§ 7-25) is correct because it is based on an eternal and infallible law of nature.

54. Allopathy has always been the dominant therapy and has expressed itself in many different systems.[60] Each system claims understandings of disease and therefore *which* wrong thing needs to be removed from a patient and *how* it should be done.[61] Classifications of disease types are made naming imaginary disease pictures and ascribing actions to medicines supposed to cure these conditions. (Hence numerous text books on Materia Medica.[62])

> F/N 60: Idle speculation and theory cannot have a place in the establishment of a science.

> F/N 61: That which has to be cured in disease is viewed as material to be expelled since no one can conceive of the dynamic effect (§ 11 note) medicines exercise upon animal organisms.

> F/N 62: And many dangerous prescriptions are administered as a result.

55. Shortly after following any of these systems the suffering of patients would increase. The public would abandon these doctors but for the palliative relief afforded from time to time and their flattering and almost instantaneous action.

Isopathy

56. By means of this palliative action (antipathic, enantiopathic) introduced seventeen centuries ago by Galen's teaching 'Contraria contrariis', physicians would gain the trust of patients by their instantaneous improvement. We shall now see how harmful this can be.[63]

F/N 63: There are those who would also like to introduce a third method, *Isopathy*, treating a disease with the identical miasm that produced it. The virus is given to the patient in a highly potentised state and therefore in an altered condition, and the cure is effected only by opposing a *simillimum* with a *simillimum*. This idea has come from the success of using cowpox as a vaccination against smallpox. But cowpox and smallpox differ in many respects, are only similar and in no way the same disease. Certain animal diseases will give us remedies for human diseases, but to use human morbific matter as a remedy for the same disease will cause trouble and aggravation.

Allopathy

57. The palliative antipathic method treats a single troublesome symptom, ignoring the many others in the disease, with a medicine which produces the exact opposite symptom, and from which can be expected the speediest, palliative relief. (Examples follow).

58. However I postulate that when medicines are used antipathically or palliatively, as above, for chronic complaints, temporary relief is always followed later by aggravation. This is explained however as being the fault of the original disease or the appearance of a new one.[64]

F/N 64: Some examples of the above observed in practice.

59. The symptoms of long-standing disease *have never* been treated in this way without a relapse occurring a few hours afterwards. (Rest of paragraph relates many examples of this statement.[65])

F/N 65: A reference to the one of the examples.

60. This is through using medicines antipathically; by prescribing a stronger dose with each new aggravation a brief transient suppression of symptoms occurs.[66] By palliating repeatedly in this way another or

an incurable condition often results. It *never* produces a *cure*.

F/N 66: A note about Brousseau and his techniques, including bleeding or venesection, with some descriptions of their effects .

61. If physicians had been capable of reflection they would have stopped repeating the poor results of antipathy and thought about the *exact opposite*. Their only successes were due to the accidental use of a medicine homœopathic to the disease.

62. The following facts explain upon what the pernicious results of the palliative, antipathic method and the efficacy of the homœopathic method depend.

Primary and Secondary Action

63. Every agent or medicine that acts upon and deranges the vital force alters the health of an individual, this is the *primary action*. The vital force reacts to maintain equilibrium, this is the *secondary action* or *counter-action*.

64. The vital force behaves in a passive or receptive way during the primary process. It then appears to rally in response and to develop:
a) the *counter-action* or *secondary action* – an opposite condition proportional to the effect of the *primary action* and the energy of the vital force; or
b) if such an opposite secondary action does not exist in nature, it will try to reassert itself, extinguish the alteration and resume normal function *(secondary action, curative action)*.

65. A number of examples of the counter-action or secondary action as explained in § 64 a) above.

66. An obvious secondary counter-action is not noticeable when minute homœopathic doses are used. They certainly produce a

primary action that is noticeable to a sufficiently attentive observer but the organism only employs against it enough secondary action as is needed to restore normal conditions.

67. The above facts which are observable in nature demonstrate the beneficial effect of homœopathic treatment and the perversity of antipathic and palliative treatment.[67]

F/N 67: Only in the most urgent cases, such as choking, drowning, poisonings, etc., where danger to life and imminent death allow us no time for the action of homœopathic remedies, is it admissible as a preliminary measure to restore sensitivity with a palliative. (Some examples follow). As long as the characteristic symptoms of disease are covered by a remedy, it does not matter if some of the smaller symptoms are actually opposite as they will disappear by themselves.

68. In homœopathic cures, after the smallest dose (see §§ 275-287) sufficient to overcome the natural disease, a slight medicinal disease is left, but so slight and mild that the vital force needs little exertion to raise the health to complete cure (§ 64 b).

Homœopathic -v- Allopathic Treatment

69. The opposite happens in antipathic, palliative treatment. An opposite medicinal symptom is chosen which touches the diseased point but only masks it for a short time from the vital principle. They dynamically neutralise[68] or remove one another. But the *opposite* cannot occupy the same place in the organism as a similar, stronger, artificial disease can. As soon as the opposite medicinal disease is extinguished it leaves the original disease as it was and, also, compels the vital force to produce an opposite condition to it. This, of course, is an analogue to the original disease and therefore compounds it.[69] The disease therefore becomes worse after the palliative has worn off.[70] The larger the dose the greater the aggravation.

F/N 68: They do not amalgamate forming a new compound as do some substances in the laboratory. Antagonistic sensations do not permanently remove one another.

F/N 69: Some say that the palliative, in its secondary action, must be capable of curing because it is similar to the disease – just as a homœopathic medicine does by its primary action. But the secondary effect is not a product of the medicine but the antagonistic reaction of the vital force. It is a state similar to the symptoms of the disease which the palliative left uneradicated. It is a reaction of the vital force against the palliative which consequently increases the symptoms still more.

F/N 70: As when in the dark a sudden light illuminates everything, but upon being extinguished leaves everything much more difficult to see.

Summary – Section 1

70. From everything said, the following truths are unmistakable:

♦ The only things to be cured in disease are the sufferings and change in health of the patient, in short the totality of symptoms. Every internal cause, occult quality or imaginary material morbific principle, is nothing but an idle dream.

♦ Health can be regained by restoring the vital force using medicines able to alter health; that is to say, produce characteristic symptoms which can be ascertained by provings on the healthy.

♦ Disease cannot be cured by medicines producing an alien morbid state *differing* from that of the disease. This does not happen in nature however strong a new dissimilar disease.

♦ Medicines producing an opposite symptom *antagonistic* to the single symptom of a disease also cannot cure but only ameliorate, then aggravate.

♦ *Homœopathy* is the third and only other possible method, in which a medicine is chosen having been proven on a healthy individual and seen to produce symptoms similar to the *totality of symptoms* of a disease. It then overpowers and extinguishes the disease by means of its similarity to it.

SECTION 2

THE TASK OF CURING

71. This being said the task of curing arrives at the following:

I   How is the physician to determine what must be known in order to cure the disease?

II How can the physician discover the pathogenic powers of the medicines?

III How to most suitably employ medicines for the cure of natural disease.

I   How Is The Physician To Determine What Must Be Known In Order To Cure The Disease?

Acutes and Chronics

72. Diseases are acute or chronic. *Acute* diseases run their course and end more or less quickly. *Chronic* diseases, often unnoticed at the beginning, untune the organism gradually in such a way that the automatic vital force only offers imperfect resistance and cannot extinguish them on its own, becoming more and more untuned until the organism dies. They are caused by dynamic contagion with a chronic miasm.

73. Acute diseases can be brought on by an individual being exposed to harmful influences such as eating excesses or privations, traumas, chill or over-heating, fatigue, etc., and also psychic upsets. Most acutes are passing flare-ups of latent psora, which return to the dormant state by themselves if not too violent and quickly eliminated. There are *sporadic* diseases brought on by harmful meteorological or telluric influences which only a few people are susceptible to at any time.

There are *epidemic* diseases in which many are affected similarly from a similar cause; in crowded areas they tend to become *contagious*. These cause characteristic fevers[71] and as they have an identical origin they set up an identical morbid process in those they affect leading to death or recovery if left untreated. War, flood and famine are often their exciting cause or breeders, and sometimes they are *acute miasms* that recur in their peculiar form, and have their established names; some are once in a lifetime, like smallpox and measles, whooping cough, red scarlet fever of Sydenham[72], mumps etc., others recur frequently like Levant plague, yellow fever, Asiatic cholera etc.

> F/N 71: The orthodox school gives different names to fevers in order to follow preconceived patterns of treatment. Homœopathy treats the characteristics of each condition according to its peculiarities.

> F/N 72: Relates a particular fever and its treatment.

Artificial/Medicinal Illnesses

74. We must include the result of artificial illness created by the prolonged use of inappropriate drugs.[73] They weaken the vital force and untune it causing it to make large changes in the organism in order to cope.[74]

> F/N 73/74: Footnotes discussing bloodletting and allopathy.

75. Bad health brought on by poor allopathic treatment is the most incurable of chronic diseases and impossible to treat with remedies once beyond a considerable point.

76. Only for natural diseases has Providence given us, through homœopathy, the means to relieve. Debilitation caused by harmful treatment[75] *must be remedied by the vital force itself* (with appropriate aid given to remove any chronic miasm in the background) provided the life

force itself is not already too weakened. This can take several years.

> F/N 75: If the patient later dies the results of harmful treatment are often explained as being due to the original disease.

Maintaining Factor Diseases

77. Diseases caused by *avoidable* influences should not be called chronic, *e.g.,* harmful food and drink, excesses, deprivation of a thing necessary to life, unhealthy places like swamps, dwelling in cellars or damp, lack of exercise and fresh air, over exertion both physical and mental, continued emotional stress. These will go away by themselves under an improved mode of living if no chronic miasm is present.

Chronic Diseases and Miasms

78. Natural, real *chronic* diseases arise from a chronic miasm and left to themselves continue to increase indefinitely despite the best habits. These are the most numerous excepting those caused by medical malpractice (§ 74). Robust constitutions, orderly living and lively vital energy are not able to eradicate them.[76]

> F/N 76: Although people may seem quite healthy, especially when young, it will inevitably be brought out in later years by adverse events or circumstances, such as debilitating passions, worry and care, and especially inappropriate medical treatment.

79. Until now only syphilis has been recognised as a chronic miasmatic disease. Sycosis has not, even though it undoubtedly is. It is thought to be cured with the destruction of the skin growths despite the lingering decline remaining.

80. More widespread and important is the chronic miasm of psora,[77] announcing itself (after the complete internal infection of the organism) through a characteristic cutaneous eruption with tickling,

itching and a specific odour sometimes consisting of a few vesicles. It is the fundamental *cause* and creator of almost all the many disease forms not due to syphilis and sycosis. (Examples follow of various forms of psoric miasmatic diseases commonly described as independent diseases.)

> F/N 77: I spent 12 years researching chronic affections and discovering the principal antipsoric remedies. I have published my observations in *The Chronic Diseases*. Up to now I could only teach how to treat chronic diseases as isolated, individual maladies according to the group of symptoms it presented, just like an idiopathic disease. Now the physician can select far more specific homœopathic remedies for chronic affections arising from psora (antipsorics) and render more essential service, and almost invariably effect a perfect cure.

81. We can begin to see how psora can be displayed in so many different disease forms if we consider the fact that psora has been passed and inherited through hundreds of generations since ancient times, and also the great number of circumstances[78] that contribute to the large variety of chronic diseases (or secondary symptoms of psora), and the divere constitutions of people affected. These have all formerly been treated under different pathological[79] names as diseases of independent character.

> F/N 78: Climate, the physical characteristics of a place, physical and mental influences of our youth, business, conditions of life, diet, passions, manners, habits and customs can all modify the transformation of psora into chronic diseases.

> F/N 79: Different epidemics are diagnosed as being one pathological condition and then treated identically because they happen to have perhaps only one symptom the same. Even if the treatment is not always identical, why make use of an

identical name which then suggests the same treatment? Each epidemic is a new disease and has never appeared in exactly the same form. It always differs in its course as well as in many of its most striking symptoms and appearance. We must not treat according to the similarity of the name of a single symptom but according to the totality of the signs of the state of each particular patient. We should only use names for diseases when explaining to ordinary people and only then to say the patient has a *kind* of dropsy... typhus... ague...etc.

82. Although the discovery of the psoric miasm and its more specific remedies helps us to understand diseases better, it is still indispensable to ascertain the symptoms and characteristics of each chronic (psoric) disease (individualisation). When investigating a case some difference is to be made if the affection is acute and rapidly developing rather than chronic, as much less time is required for tracing the picture of the disease and fewer questions need to be asked. The main symptoms tend to be more obvious and the history of the disease is obviously shorter and easier to ascertain[80] than in a chronic disease of many years standing.

F/N 80: Therefore the following directions for investigating the symptoms are only partially applicable for acute diseases.

Taking the Case

83. In this individualising *examination of a case of disease* the practitioner must bear in mind only what is applicable for each individual case. Be *free from prejudice* and attentive in observation, and trace carefully the picture of the disease.

84. The patient will relate his case, and friends and relatives will tell us about his behaviour, complaints and everything they have noticed in him. The physician sees, hears and observes with his other senses what

has been altered in, and is peculiar to, the patient. He writes all this down exactly as related by both patient and relations, especially their verbatim expressions. As long as they do not unduly digress he lets them talk without interruption[81] as this disturbs their train of thought. At the beginning ask them to speak slowly so we can write down the important parts of what they say.

> F/N 81: Every interruption breaks the train of thought and often what they would have said at first does not occur to them again in precisely the same way.

85. Write down every new circumstance mentioned on a fresh line so that all symptoms appear separately. They can then be added to later if subsequently more explicitly explained.

86. When finished talking read over the symptoms again as they were related to you, one by one. Then ask for more precise information on each symptom: *e.g.,* when did the symptom occur? Was it previous to taking the medicine? While taking the medicine? After stopping the medicine? What kind of pain, and the exact sensation? Where exactly? How often did the pain occur and at what times? In fits or by itself? Or continued without intermission? How long did it last? At what time of the day or night and in what position of the body was it worse or ceased entirely? What was the exact nature of the circumstances - described in plain language?

87. Then we will obtain precise information. This should be done without putting words into the patient's mouth[82] or by asking questions that can be answered 'yes' or 'no', thereby illiciting half truths or untruths, or denials to avoid discomfort. A false picture of the disease and an unsuitable treatment would result.

> F/N 82: Do not ask if some particular circumstance was present. Never be guilty of making suggestions which tend to

seduce the patient into giving false answers.

88. If nothing has been mentioned about several other functions of the body or his mental state then ask.[83] But only use general expressions so that the patient or attendants are forced to supply all the specific details.

> F/N 83: For example: what are the stools like? How does he pass water? How is his day and night sleep? What is his mood like his humour, memory? How about thirst? What sort of taste does he have in his mouth? What food and drinks are desired? Or aversions? Do they taste natural or have some unusual taste? What about the head, limbs, abdomen?

89. When the patient (we must rely on the patient for a description of his sensations, except in feigned diseases) has given us all this information freely of his own accord and traced a tolerably perfect picture of the disease, ask more precise questions[84] if you feel you have not gained all the information needed.

> F/N 84: For example: how often are the bowels moved? What is the exact character of the stools? Did the whitish evacuation consist of mucus or fæces? Were there pains during the evacuation? What was their character and where? What did the patient vomit? Is the bad taste in the mouth putrid, bitter, sour, or what? Before, during or after eating? When was it worse? What is the taste of the eructation? Does the urine only become thick when left standing, or when first passed? What is the colour when first passed? What colour is the sediment? How does he behave during sleep? Does he whine, moan, talk, cry out or start during sleep? Does he snore during inspiration or expiration? Does he lie on his back or on which side? Does he cover up well or cannot bear clothes? Does he awake easily or sleep too soundly? How does he feel immediately after waking

from sleep? How often do the symptoms occur? Does it come on while sitting, lying, standing, in motion, when fasting, in the morning, evening, after a meal, or when does it appear? When did the rigor come on? Was it a chilly sensation or was he actually cold at the same time? If so, in what parts? Or while feeling chilly was he actually warm to the touch? Was it merely a sensation of cold without shivering or was he hot without redness of the face? What parts of him were hot to the touch? Or did he complain of heat without being hot to the touch? How long did the chilliness last? How long was the hot stage? When did the thirst come on – during the cold stage? During the heat? Or previous to it? Or subsequent to it? How large was the thirst and what was desired? When did the sweat come on – at the beginning or the end of the heat? Or how many hours after the heat? When asleep or when awake? How great was the sweat? Was it warm or cold? On what parts? How did it smell? What does he complain of before or during the cold stage, or hot stage? Or after it? Or during or after the sweating stage? In women, note the character of menstruation and other discharges, etc.

90. After writing down these statements record what you observe in the patient[85] and determine how much was peculiar to the patient in his healthy state.

F/N 85: For example: how did the patient behave during the visit? Was he morose, quarrelsome, hasty, tearful, anxious, despairing, sad, hopeful, calm, etc? Was he in a drowsy state or dull of comprehension? Did he speak hoarsely, or in a low tone, or incoherently, or how else? What was the colour of his face and eyes and skin generally? What degree of liveliness and power was in the expression and eyes? What was the tongue like, his breathing, the smell from his mouth, and hearing? Were the pupils dilated or contracted? How rapidly and to what extent did they alter in the light and dark? What was the character of the pulse? The condition of the abdomen? How moist or hot, cold or dry to the touch was the skin of this or that part – or generally? Was he lying with the head thrown back, with mouth fully or half open, with the arms placed above the head, on his back, or in what position? What effort did he make to raise himself? And anything else that may strike you as being remarkable.

Considering the Case – Medicines that Mask Symptoms

91. After a course of unsuitable medicine you will not observe a true disease picture. However, symptoms and complaints *before taking the medicines or several days after discontinuing them* will give the true fundamental idea of the *original* form of the disease. These must be especially recorded. If the disease is chronic and the patient is still taking medicine, he should be left without medicine for a few days or given something non-medicinal, postponing detailed examination of the case.

92. If, however, the disease is rapidly developing and serious we must consider it as it is; even if it is altered by medicines and the original symptom picture is not evident. We will then be faced with the medicinal disease combined with the original disease, which will generally be graver for the use of inappropriate drugs, and therefore demanding prompt and efficient attention.

Considering the Case – Causes of Disease

93. If the disease was caused by something obvious, either recently, or in the case of a chronic disease, some time ago, then the patient or his friends will either mention it spontaneously or when carefully questioned.[86]

F/N 86: If the cause is of a disgraceful character we must learn to elicit the information by skilful questioning. The following causes are usually of this nature: poisoning or attempted suicide, masturbation, debauchery, alcoholism, coffee, over eating generally or with some specific food, venereal diseases, disappointed love, jealousy, domestic infelicity, worry, grief on account of some family misfortune, ill-usage, frustrated revenge, injured pride, financial embarrassment, superstitious fear, hunger, imperfection in the private parts, a rupture, prolapse, and so on.

94. In a chronic disease find out about the patient's usual occupations, mode of living, diet, domestic situation and so forth, to see if there is anything producing or maintaining the disease. Its removal will promote recovery.[87]

> F/N 87: In the chronic diseases of women it is especially necessary to pay attention to pregnancy, sterility, sexual desire, births, miscarriages, suckling, and the state of the period. With respect to the period find out if it occurs at too short intervals or is delayed, its duration, whether the flow is continuous or interrupted, the general quantity, how dark the colour is, whether there is leucorrhœa before or afterwards, but especially by what bodily or mental ailments, sensations and pain, it is preceded with, accompanied or followed. If there is leucorrhœa, what is its nature, what sensations attend its flow, how much is there and what are the conditions and occasions under which it occurs?

95. In chronic cases, as well as investigating the signs of disease as mentioned above, pay careful attention to the most minute peculiarities. This is partly because they are the most characteristic and least resemble those of acute diseases, and partly because patients grow used to prolonged suffering and pay no attention to small accessory symptoms which are often characteristic. They almost consider them

natural having forgotten real health and don't think they are connected with the chief complaint.

96. Patients differ so much in their dispositions. Some, especially so-called hypochondriacs and other sensitives, present symptoms too vividly and use exaggerated expressions to encourage the physician to help them.[88]

> F/N 88: Even the most extreme hypochondriac will not fabricate symptoms. We must make allowances for their exaggerations which should be seen as an important symptom. The insane and rascals who fabricate their diseases are a different matter.

97. There are patients of an opposite character who keep back their complaints, either from laziness, modesty, mildness or backwardness. They describe them in vague terms or allege they are of no consequence.

98. We need to listen to the patient's story and give credence to his own expressions because friends and relatives will always alter things a little when reporting an illness. Even more so, and especially in chronic diseases we need a special circumspection, tact, knowledge of human nature, caution and patience when taking the case.

99. Taking the cases of acutes and recent chronic diseases are the easiest, as health is a recent phenomenon in the mind of the patient and friends. We certainly need to know just as much in such cases, but there is less to *inquire into* as they are usually spontaneously related to us.

Epidemics

100. In epidemic and sporadic diseases it does not matter if something with the same name has appeared before. We must take the pure picture of each prevailing disease as if it were something new and

unknown. Careful examination will show that every prevailing disease differs vastly from all previous epidemics. The only exceptions are those epidemics caused by a contagious principle that always remains the same such as smallpox, measles, etc.

101. It may easily happen that in the first case seen in an epidemic we do not discover the complete picture. It is only on close observation of several cases that we see the totality of the epidemic's signs and symptoms. If carefully observant we can, however, after only one or two patients, arrive at a true picture and even succeed in finding a suitable remedy.

102. From writing down the symptoms of several cases the disease picture becomes more complete. General symptoms (*e.g.,* loss of appetite, sleeplessness, etc.) become precisely defined and special symptoms, which are peculiar to few diseases and occur more rarely, become prominent and constitute what is characteristic of a malady.[89] People catching an epidemic at the same time have the *same* disease from the same source, but we have to see several patients of differing constitutions to record the totality of its symptoms.

> F/N 89: If we have been able to choose a remedy for the first cases we will be able to verify its suitability or find a more appropriate remedy from the later cases.

Miasms

103. I have applied the same method for epidemics to miasmatic chronic diseases, which always remain the same in their essential nature, especially psora. The whole sphere of their symptoms must be investigated, as a patient only manifests a portion of the miasmatic chronic disease's symptoms. Other patients will exhibit other symptoms, which again are also only a portion of the whole. The whole nature of a miasmatic chronic disease (especially psora) can only be seen from observing *many* single patients affected with it. Only

then will we be able to find those remedies capable of curing – the antipsorics. These medicines are the true remedies of the many patients suffering from such chronic affections.

104. When the totality of symptoms or picture of the disease (of whatever kind) is accurately sketched,[90] the most difficult part of the task is done. We can then pick out the characteristic symptoms and choose a remedy. And then, at a subsequent examination, in order to see the effect of the remedy and the change in the patient's state, we can strike out the symptoms that have been ameliorated, mark what remain, and add any new symptoms that may have occured.

> F/N 90: The old school doctor paid little attention to the minute details in a case, and wrote prescriptions composed of ingredients, the true effect of which were unknown to him. (A description follows of the old school doctors' mode of operation and the invariably bad results thereof).

II   How Can The Physician Discover The Pathogenic Powers Of The Medicines?

The Argument for Provings

105. We must acquire an understanding of the power of the remedies, or *instruments of cure,* in order to select a remedy which can produce an artificial disease as similar as possible to the natural disease needing to be cured.

106. We must know the entire pathogenic action of several remedies – all the disease symptoms and alterations in health they can cause in the healthy individual – before we can hope to select suitable remedies for most of the natural diseases.

107. We cannot test the effect of remedies on *sick* people as the

symptoms would be mixed up with the symptoms of their natural diseases.

108. There is no better way of discovering what disease symptoms remedies are able to produce, than by giving them to *healthy* people and subsequently noting the changes, symptoms and signs in body and mind[91] (see §§ 24-27).

> F/N 91: As far as I know only Albrecht von Haller has seen the necessity of testing medicines in this way other than myself.

109. It is only through homœopathy[92] that the certain cure of human maladies is possible.[93]

> F/N 92: He goes on to justify this claim.

> F/N 93: References to some of Hahnemann's articles.

110. The reports of poisonings with various medicines correspond with provings on myself and other healthy individuals with the same remedies. It never occured to the authors of these reports that they were revealing the power of the drugs to cure disease.[94]

> F/N 94: See *Examination of the Sources of the Ordinary Materia Medica* – prefix of the 3rd part *Materia Medica Pura,* vol ii.

111. This correspondence between poisonings and provings convinces me that medicines act *according to fixed, eternal laws of nature* and produce *certain, reliable disease symptoms, each according to its own peculiar character.*

112. One also sees in these old reports states appearing at the end of a poisoning opposite in nature to those that first appeared. These symptoms are the reverse of the *primary action* (§ 63) of the medicines

on the vital force. They are the reaction of the vital force – the *secondary action* (§§ 62-67). One hardly ever sees this secondary action with moderate doses and never with small doses. In the homœopathic cure the organism only reacts as much as is necessary to regain health (§ 67).

113. Only narcotic medicines seem to be an exception. In their primary action they sometimes take away sensation, sensitivity and irritability. In their *secondary action* they often increase sensitivity and irritability, even in moderate doses on healthy people.

114. Excepting narcotics, in experiments with moderate doses of medicine on healthy people we only see the primary action at work.

115. In some medicines you will sometimes see symptoms occurring which are directly opposite to previous or subsequent symptoms. These are not the *secondary action* of the vital force but are alternating states in various paroxysms of the primary action. These are called *alternating actions.*

116. Some symptoms are frequently produced by the medicines in a lot of people, other symptoms more rarely or in a few people, some symptoms only in very few people.

117. The symptoms produced in only very few people are called *idiosyncrasies,* by which is meant constitutions which are healthy but tend to be brought into a more or less morbid state by things which *seem* to produce no effect in many other people.[95] But this absence of effect on everyone is only *apparent;* two things are necessary to produce symptoms:- the power of the influencing substance and the susceptibility to it of the vital force. With idiosyncrasies everyone must be affected, otherwise the same substances would not work as medicines on *all* sick people.[96]

F/N 95: A few people are apt to faint from the smell of roses, or become sick from eating mussels, crabs and the roe of the Barbel, or from touching the leaves of some plants.

F/N 96: A case where someone who fainted was restored by rose water and another where rose vinegar was of use in the same condition.

118. Every medicine will exhibit peculiar actions on an organism which are not produced by any other medicine in exactly the same way.[97]

F/N 97: A. v. Haller saw this when he said, "A great diversity of strength lies hidden in these plants themselves, whose external features we have long known but whose souls, as it were, and whatever divine element they have, we have not yet perceived."

119. Every plant and mineral salt is different in its external and inner form and growth. In the same way they differ in their pathogenetic and curative properties.[98] Each will alter the health of humans in a different and determinate manner.[99]

F/N 98: If we know the different effects of each remedy we will appreciate that one medicine cannot prove as serviceable as another in a disease. There are no equivalent remedies, no *surrogates*.

F/N 99: We cannot employ any remedy in a disease except one tested on the healthy and known to be more similar than any other to the disease to be cured.

120. Therefore medicines must be carefully distinguished from one another by being tested on the healthy through careful experiment. Then we can learn their power and real effect and treat disease with their correct selection.

Provings

121. In proving medicines upon the healthy remember strong substances are liable, even in small doses, to produce changes in health, even the health of robust people. Milder substances must be given in larger doses. To observe the action of the very weakest medicines they should be tested on healthy people who are delicate, irritable and sensitive, and free from disease.

122. In these experiments only use medicines of whose purity, genuineness and energy we are sure. The exactitude of future medicine depends upon this.

123. Any medicine must be taken in a simple and unadulterated form. Mix the fresh juice from indigenous plants with a little alcohol (rectified wine spirit equivalent to 95 degree grain alcohol – see § 270); exotic plants, in the form of powder or tincture prepared with alcohol (wine spirit) when they are fresh, with water; salts and gums, however, should be dissolved in water just before being taken. If you can only obtain the plant in a dried state and its powers are naturally weak, make an infusion by cutting the herb into small pieces and pouring boiling water on it, then take it immediately while still warm, otherwise, without any alcohol the medicinal powers will be lost.

124. Every medicine should be proved alone and in perfect purity without any other substances added or taken at the same time, for as long as the experiment and observation lasts.

125. The diet should be regulated, nutritious and simple, and free from spices during the proving. Avoid green vegetables,[100] roots, salads, and herb soups. Drinks should be those usually taken and as little stimulating as possible.[101]

> F/N 100: Young green peas, green french beans, boiled potatoes and carrots are allowable.

F/N 101: Provers should not be in the habit of drinking wine, brandy, coffee or tea, or must totally abstain for a considerable period before the proving.

126. The prover should avoid all mental and physical over-exertions, and dissipating passions. He should have no urgent business distractions, be able to devote himself to careful observation, be of sound health and possess enough intelligence to define and describe his sensations accurately.

127. Provers must be both male and female to reveal alterations to health in the sexual sphere.

128. Potentised medicines will disclose more about their properties than in their crude state. Even substances considered inert are called into activity by potentisation through trituration and succussion. The prover should take 4-6 very small globules daily, on an empty stomach, of the 30th potency for several days, moistened with a little water or dissolved in water and thoroughly mixed.

129. If only slight effects appear then several additional pellets may be taken until their effects become perceptible. Drugs do not exert equal strength upon everyone. A delicate personality may be strongly affected by a weak drug and hardly at all by a strong drug. Or a robust person may be strongly affected by a weak drug and very slightly from a strong one. As this is not to be predetermined it is advisable that each prover should begin with a small dose gradually increased as necessary.

130. If we have given a sufficiently strong dose at the beginning of an experiment, we have the advantage of the prover learning the exact consecutive order in which the symptoms appear, and noting the times each occured. This helps show the distinct order in which primary and alternating actions appear. A small dose will often suffice providing the

experimenter is sensitive and pays proper attention to the state of his sensations. The duration of the action of a drug can be seen after comparing a number of experiments.

131. We might need to increase dosage to gain an effect, in which case, although we may discover the various morbid conditions the drug produces (but not the consecutive order of their appearance), the second dose may by its curative effect often remove some of the symptoms or produce an opposite state. These symptoms should be enclosed in brackets until other exact experiments show whether they are the secondary action (of the organism) or an alternating action of the medicine.

132. But if we want to observe the symptoms of a medicine without reference to their order of appearance or duration of action (especially a weak medicine), it is better to give a dose for several days, increasing the dose every day. This is how the action of an unknown medicine, even a mild one, is revealed especially if tested on sensitive people.

133. When a sensation appears the prover should assume various postures to determine the exact character of the symptom, *e.g.,* moving the affected part, walking in the room or in the open air, standing, sitting, lying (see if it returns when assuming the original position), eating, drinking, talking, coughing, sneezing or other bodily functions. Also note the time of day or night at which the symptom appears.

134. Not all the symptoms of a remedy will manifest in the same person, or at the same time. A prover will experience certain symptoms in one trial, and others during a second and third trial. Symptoms seen in the fourth prover may not be seen again until the eighth or tenth person. They also may not recur at the same hour.

135. The totality of a drug is only seen by many provings on a variety

of people of both sexes. We should not consider the proving complete until all provers are not observing any new symptoms and see mostly symptoms already experienced by others.

136. Although a medicine cannot produce all of its symptoms in one person, the tendency to do so nevertheless exists (§ 17) and is brought into operation in the case of every individual when ill and presenting similar symptoms. It then cures through the law of similars, being homœopathically selected.

137. The more moderate the dose (within certain limits) selected for proving, the more distinctly appear the primary effects without being mixed with the counter effects of the vital force. If excessively large doses are used some secondary symptoms will occur and the primary effects will come on in such hurried confusion that they will be difficult to observe accurately. This can also create a danger to the prover.

138. If the above conditions are adhered to (§§ 124-127), all deviations from normal health must be ascribed to the medicine, even if symptoms reappear that a prover suffered from in the past. Their reappearance shows that the prover is disposed to such symptoms being excited in him. They are produced by the drug. Symptoms do not appear spontaneously but are produced by the medicine.

139. The prover should write down all sensations, sufferings, accidents and changes in health at the time they occur, the time elapsed before the symptoms occurred, as well as the duration of the symptoms. The physician should examine the report at the termination of the experiment or, if over several days, examine the prover daily, questioning the exact form of every symptom while fresh in the memory.[102]

F/N 102: The author of such provings is responsible for the

trustworthiness of the prover and his statements.

140. If the prover cannot write, the physician must interview him or her everyday. He should obtain the voluntary statements of the prover as far as possible. He should not guess or extort statements (§§ 84-99).

141. The best provings are those *done by the sensitive physician upon himself*.[103]

> F/N 103: A physician will become a better observer and need not fear the slight ailments caused by the medicines. On the contrary the prover's organism becomes more expert at repelling external morbific influences.

142. Distinguishing symptoms[104] produced by a medicine, from those of a disease it was taken to cure, (especially of a chronic character) is very difficult and should be left to expert observers.

> F/N 104: Symptoms observed either in the distant past or not at all, and therefore new and belonging to the medicine.

Materia Medica

143. After many drugs have been tested carefully we will then possess a true and reliable[105] materia medica. It will contain a record of artificial morbid states.

> F/N 105: Lately it has been the habit to pay unknown persons at distant locations as provers. The results lose all value due to lack of greatest moral certainty and trustworthiness.

144. The materia medica should exclude conjecture, assertion and imagination and contain the pure language of nature in response to careful enquiry.

145. It is necessary to have a large materia medica in order to address all the many disease conditions in the world.[106] Even now few diseases remain for which a homœopathic remedy may not be found.[107]

> F/N 106: Numbers of *accurate and trustworthy* observers need to enrich the only true materia medica by careful *experiments on themselves*. The healing art will then approach the mathematical sciences in certainty.

> F/N: 107: See the second note to § 109.

III How To Most Suitably Employ Medicines For The Cure Of Natural Disease

Curing Disease

146. *The third point* of the duty of the true physician relates to the application of the *medicines in order to homœopathically cure diseases.* (§§ 72 and 105)

147. A tested drug most similar to a disease will cure it.

148. Repeat of the description of how a homœopathic remedy works. In acute diseases after the administration of the correct remedy a disease will disappear if recently developed, in a few hours. Older chronic diseases will take longer by using several doses of the same remedy or careful selection[108] of several.

> F/N 108: This laborious search for the most suitable remedy demands much deliberation. The most suitable homœopathic remedy does not fly into our mouths like roasted pigeons. The argument continues against the 'new mongrel sect' who give an unsuitable homœopathic remedy at the same time as an

allopathic remedy and blame the homœopathic principle for their failure.

General Points

149. Old chronic diseases, especially if complicated by allopathic medicines which rob the patient of strength, require more time for cure.

150. One or more recent, trifling symptoms are not a disease and can often be removed by a change of diet or mode of living.

151. If the symptoms are few and severe, enquiry will generally discover several other symptoms of less severity which will complete the picture of the case.

152. If an acute disease is severe the symptoms will be clear and numerous and increase the certainty of finding a remedy providing we possess a sufficient number of well recorded medicines.

Finding a Remedy

153. We search for a remedy by comparing the totality of symptoms of the disease with the list of symptoms of our tested drugs. The *more striking, singular, uncommon and peculiar* symptoms[109] should bear the closest similitude to the desired medicine. The more general and undefined the symptom the less important, as they are observed in almost every disease and drug.

> F/N 109: Drs. von Boenninghausen and Jahr have rendered a great service by the publishing of their books on characteristic and principal symptoms.

154. If the chosen remedy has the peculiar, uncommon and characteristic symptoms in the greatest number and similarity to the

disease, then *this* medicine is the most homœopathic for *this* disease and will cure, generally by one dose in a recent disease without any considerable disturbance.

155. *Without any considerable disturbance* means that only those symptoms of the medicine similar to the disease are activated. Symptoms belonging to the remedy but having no affinity will remain quiescent. We see little of them because of the minuteness of the dosage.

156. However, one can always expect to see at least one unusual sensation or slight new symptom if the dosage is not sufficiently small in susceptible patients. But this is easily compensated for by the activity of the organism and is often not noticed by the average patient. Recovery will take place as long as their are no heterogenous medicinal influences or excesses.

Aggravations

157. The remedy will, in the first hour or in a few hours, produce a slight aggravation resembling the acute disease. A dose that is too large may cause a longer aggravation but this is a *medicinal disease* stronger than the original affection, even though to the patient it may seem to be an aggravation of the disease.

158. A slight *homœopathic aggravation* in the first hours is a very good prognostic that the acute disease will yield to the first dose. The drug disease must be more intense to overcome the natural disease. (See §§ 43-48)

159. The smaller the dose in acute diseases the smaller and shorter the aggravation during the first hours.

160. We cannot reduce the remedy dosage so much that it cannot

overcome the disease. Therefore we must expect the appropriate medicine to produce a perceptible aggravation during the first hour after its ingestion.[110]

> F/N 110: This has been noticed by other physicians who have accidently employed a homœopathic remedy. An increase of the itch after treatment with Sulphur is readily assumed to be an increase of the itch but it is in fact a Sulphur eruption. Two examples of similar cases follow in the footnote.

161. Homœopathic aggravations (or the primary effect of the remedy intensifying the symptoms of the original disease) occurring in a few hours, belong to acutes or diseases of recent origin. In long-standing diseases no aggravations should be allowed to appear during treatment, and they do not appear if the chosen remedy was given in proper small, gradually higher doses (see § 247). The aggravation of the original symptoms often appear only at the end of treatment when the cure is almost or quite finished.

162. Until we have many more drugs at our disposal we may have to resort to a less than perfect curative agent that only covers a *portion* of the symptoms.

163. In this case a perfect and easy cure cannot then be expected as disturbances will follow that were not previously encountered in the disease; accessory symptoms of the not perfectly appropriate remedy. This does not prevent a considerable part of the disease being eradicated and thereby commencing a cure. But the accessory symptoms are always mild if the dose is sufficiently minute.

164. Cure will follow without any particular disturbance *when these few medicinal symptoms are mainly uncommon and peculiarly characteristic of the disease.*

Suspect Prescriptions

165. But if the remedy has no characteristic, peculiar or uncommon symptoms of accurate similitude to the disease and corresponds by general and vaguely defined symptoms, and among the known medicines there are none more homœopathically appropriate, then we can expect little result.

166. This will be *rare* owing to the recent addition of well tested remedies. If it should occur then the delay will be short as soon as a medicine of more striking similitude is selected.

167. If, in an acute case, this wrong remedy produces strong accessory symptoms, its dose should not be allowed to complete its action. Re-examine and consider the remaining original symptoms and new ones as a new picture of the disease.

168. If the remedy then given is insufficient to completely destroy the disease, examine again the remaining morbid condition and select another remedy. Repeat this process until the patient is healthy.

169. Because of limited remedies, cases occur which we cannot cover by one remedy. We find one half of the symptoms covered by one and the other half by another. Give the most suitable remedy first, but do not prescribe the other remedy without re-examining the case as it may not be indicated after the case has been changed by the action of the first remedy. Certainly, do not give both together (see note § 272). Re-take the case and prescribe according to the new set of symptoms appearing on re-examination.

170. In any case, where symptoms have changed we must re-record the case and select a remedy without regard to the second best medicine. However, if the second best remedy is still indicated (which is not often the case) then we can use it with confidence.

Repeating Remedies

171. In non-venereal psoric originated diseases we may often have to use several antipsoric remedies in succession, each selected homœopathically on symptoms left after each preceding remedy has terminated its action.

Scarcity of Symptoms - One-sided Diseases

172. *Scarcity of symptoms presented* by the disease is another problem. Removing this removes nearly all the difficulties.

173. Diseases with few symptoms, which are therefore less susceptible to cure, can be termed *one-sided* diseases. They have just one or two prominent symptoms which obscure the rest of the disease. Most of them are chronic diseases.

174. Their chief symptoms may be internal or external. The latter are more commonly called *local diseases.*

175. One sided, internal diseases which do not have enough symptoms are often due to the physician's error, having not fully discovered the symptoms present.

176. However some diseases will only exhibit one or two violent, severe symptoms despite careful investigation, (§§ 84-98) all the others being indistinct.

177. This is a *rare* occurence, but in the first place select the most homœopathic remedy based on these few symptoms.

178. Sometimes this remedy will cure, especially when the symptoms are striking, uncommon and characteristic.

179. But usually the first remedy will be only partially appropriate due

to the lack of symptoms guiding us to an accurate selection.

180. Here this partially analogous remedy (see § 162 *et seq*) will produce accessory symptoms during its action, mixing its own symptoms with the economy of the patient. *However these symptoms do belong to the disease although not previously clearly perceived,* their having been brought out by the remedy.

181. They should not be ascribed only to the remedy, even though it is true they originated from it.[111] *This* medicine needed *this* certain kind of organism to give rise to these symptoms. Therefore the new totality of symptoms must be regarded and treated as the disease itself.

> F/N 111: When they are not caused by an error in life style, violent emotions, or a strong change in health such as the occurrence or cessation of menses, conception, childbirth and so on.

Second Prescription

182. So the imperfect selection of the remedy, almost inevitable due to the lack of symptoms, completes the picture of the disease and facilitates the discovery of a second, more accurate, remedy.

183. Whenever the dose of the first medicine ceases its beneficial effect, re-examine the case and select the next remedy accordingly, unless the newly developed symptoms are grave and demand speedier aid (excessively rare in very chronic disease due to the minuteness of homœopathic remedies). It will be all the more accurate as the group of symptoms will have become larger and more complete.[112]

> F/N: 112: When the patient is very ill (usually in acute illnesses) and the symptoms are indistinct due to the nerves being benumbed not allowing pain or suffering, this torpor can be removed by Opium. In its secondary action the symptoms of

the disease become apparent.

184. After each new dose of medicine has completed its effect and is no longer suitable and helpful the case should be re-examined to see what symptoms remain, and the most suitable remedy selected according to those symptoms, and so on until recovery is complete.

Local Affections

185. *Local affections* or diseases of external parts of the body are common in one-sided or partial diseases. They are not independent of the rest of the body and should be treated as part of the whole.

186. Recent local conditions due to injury would at first appear to merit being called *local* diseases. However if significant they affect the whole organism causing fevers etc. They often need surgical skills in order to cure, *e.g.*, in dislocations, stitches, hæmorrhages, effusions, fractures, withdrawing foreign bodies etc., though frequently *dynamic* treatment is required in order to accomplish the work of healing.

187. But external affections not caused by injury or only by a slight wound (which provided the exciting cause), are produced by an internal morbid state and it is absurd to treat these surgically.

188. These were considered *local* diseases separate from the general organism.[113]

F/N 113: One of the many blunders of the old school.

189. It is obvious that no external affection (not caused by an external injury) can originate without participation of the organism. The parts are so connected that even a lip eruption or whitlow cannot occur without previous and simultaneous internal ill-health.

190. Treatment should therefore be applied to the whole system in

order to cure such external, non-injurious affections.

191. Experience shows that an internal medicine brings about changes in the general condition and in the local, so called, isolated affection. The most wholesome effects are seen when health is restored to the whole body and external affections disappear without the use of external medication, provided the internal remedy is suitably homœopathic.

192. This is best done by selecting a remedy which covers the local affection and general condition (perhaps noticed before the use of unsuitable medicines) based on the totality of symptoms.

193. This internal medicine removes the general morbid state of the body along with the local affection, proving that the local affection depended upon the whole organism.

194. It is not beneficial in acute local diseases or local affections to rub in or apply externally a remedy as a local application when the remedy is being used internally, even if it is specific and curative. Acute local diseases brought about by internal causes will usually yield rapidly to internal remedies prescribed on the internal and external symptoms. But if a remnant of the disease is left in the affected part or the general system, the local disease often proves to be a product of psora, lain dormant, which is now about to become an actual chronic disease.

195. These cases are not uncommon and to thoroughly cure, after the acute condition has pretty well subsided, we must institute appropriate antipsoric treatment (See *Chronic Diseases*) to remove the symptoms that remain, and the morbid state of health to which the patient was previously subject. Antipsoric internal treatment is required in non-venereal chronic local disorders.

196. One may think a cure can be accelerated by using the correct

homœopathic remedy externally as well as internally.

197. But this is inadmissible in local affections not only arising from psora, but also from sycosis and syphilis and results in disadvantages. *In diseases whose chief symptom is a constant local affection, if we simultaneously apply the remedy locally and internally* the local symptoms[114] are usually annihilated more quickly than the internal disease, giving the impression of a cure and making it difficult and sometimes impossible to see if the total disease has been destroyed.

> F/N 114: Recent itch eruptions, chancre, condyloma, as indicated in *Chronic Diseases.*

198. For the same reason, we should not use medicines capable of curing internally *only* on the local symptom. If the chief, local symptom disappears, the less distinguishable symptoms that remain are less constant than the local disease; their peculiarities and characteristics are too indistinct to furnish a clear picture of the disease.

199. If the correct remedy has not been discovered[115] before the local symptoms have been destroyed by surgery or external remedies, the case becomes much more difficult as we are left with indefinite, uncharacteristic symptoms and deprived of that feature of the case which would have determined the selection of a remedy, namely the external principal symptom.

> F/N 115: As was the case before my time with remedies for condylomas and psoras.

200. If the main symptom is present, the remedy for the whole disease can be found, and if it persists it will prove the incompleteness of the cure. But if it disappears, we would then have proof that the disease is completely eradicated.

201. The vital force, when not able to overcome a disease, forms a local disease in order to silence the internal disease without curing it.[116] The local disease is a part of the general disease developed in one direction, transported to a less dangerous position. However the internal disease increases constantly which aggravates the local condition.

> F/N 116: The fontanelles of the old school physician have a similar effect. As artificial ulcers upon external parts they silence some internal chronic complaints but only for a short time without curing them. In fact they weaken and ruin the entire state of health much more than the metastases effected by the vital force.

202. When the local disease is destroyed by external remedies nature compensates by increasing the internal disease and other latent symptoms. This is usually *incorrectly* defined as the whole disease being *driven back* into the system.

203. Every external treatment of such local symptoms without curing the inner miasmatic disease, is the most prolific source of chronic diseases and one of the most criminal procedures the medical world can be guilty of; and yet it is still taught and adopted as the only one.[117]

> F/N 117: Any medicines given internally at the same time also serve to aggravate the malady as they possess no power of curing the whole disease but instead weaken the organism and inflicted other chronic medicinal diseases.

Miasms

204. By placing into one class diseases arising from bad habits (§ 77) with those caused by persistent drugging (§ 74) we shall then find all others are caused by the three chronic miasms, syphilis, sycosis and

chiefly psora. Each of these infections possessed the entire organism before the appearance of the local primary symptom of each of them (psora - scabious eruption, syphilis - the chancre or bubo, sycosis - the condylomata) that prevented their outburst. If this local symptom is removed these chronic miasmatic diseases will burst forth into an incredible number of chronic diseases, as they have done for thousands of years. (See note to § 282).

205. The homœopath does not treat one of these primary symptoms of, or secondary affections developed from, a chronic miasm by local remedies (dynamically[118] or mechanically), but cures the fundamental miasm together with the primary and secondary symptoms. However as most primary symptoms[119] will have been suppressed he must do more with the secondary symptoms, *i.e.*, the chronic diseases arising from psora.

> F/N 118: If the local problem is removed the internal disease still exists and will metastasise to a new and usually more life threatening location. Such removal will only succeed when tumours etc. are still small and the vital force is still energetic. But this is exactly the time when complete internal cure is still practicable through the use of homœopathy. Death is hastened when a cancer of the breast (for instance) is removed surgically.

> F/N 119: Itch eruption, chancre. condylomata.

More Case Taking

206. Before beginning chronic treatment carefully find out[120] if the patient has had syphilis or gonorrhœa; in which case the treatment must be directed towards this alone. When such infections have previously occurred bear it in mind in cases where psora is present because the latter will be complicated with the former. Psora is the *most frequent fundamental cause of chronic diseases*. Sometimes both psora and syphilis may be complicated with sycosis.

F/N 120: Do not take any notice in these cases when patients tell you, even in the severest diseases, that they are ill because of catching cold, or through a vexation, a sprain etc. A *healthy organism* does not develop long-term chronic ailments for these reasons. The assigned causes only rouse the latent chronic miasm.

207. Then ask what allopathic treatment and which medicines have been used, and what mineral baths (and their effects), in order to understand the degeneration of the disease from its original state, and to correct, where possible, these artificial operations, and to avoid using medicines already improperly used.

208. Then the patient's age, habits, diet, occupations, domestic circumstances and social position should be considered to see their effect on the disease and whether they might impede a cure. Also observe the state of mind and temperament to see whether it is necessary to modify anything.

209. After this is done endeavour in repeated conversations to trace the disease as completely as possible. Mark the peculiar and characteristic symptoms. Guided by these we should then select the first antipsoric, or other remedy to begin the treatment.

Temperament – Mental & Emotional Symptoms

210. One-sided diseases belong to psora and are the most difficult to cure due to this partial development – symptoms being obscured by the one prominent symptom. So called *mental diseases* are of this kind. These are not a class of disease separated from all others because the state of mind is *always* altered[121] in physical diseases and should be noted in order to trace an accurate picture of the disease.

F/N 121: Often a patient's disposition will become the opposite after treatment; mild softness becomes ingratitude, cruelty and malice; patience becomes obstinacy; chasteness, lasciviousness; clear-headedness, obtuseness.

211. The state of mind and temperament often chiefly determines the selection of the remedy, being a decidedly characteristic symptom and obvious to the accurately observing physician.

212. It is the principal feature of all diseases. All medicines can notably alter the mind and emotions of a prover and each one does so in a different way.

213. A treatment would not be according to nature (that is to say homœopathic) if we did not recognise the changes in mind and temper in both acute and chronic diseases and select a remedy which is not only similar to the physicals but also has a similar effect upon the mind and disposition.[122]

> F/N 122: Thus Aconite will seldom or *never* cure in a patient with a quiet disposition, Nux Vomica will never be useful in the mild and phlegmatic, or Pulsatilla where it is happy, gay and obstinate, or Ignatia where it is imperturbable and disposed neither to be frightened nor vexed.

Mental Diseases

214. Mental diseases should be treated like all others and are only curable by a similar remedy.

215. Most so-called diseases of the mind are really bodily diseases in which certain mental and emotional symptoms peculiar to each of them are increased. These develop, while the bodily symptoms decline, and are finally transferred like a one-sided local disease into the invisible, subtle organs of the mind.

216. Cases are not rare when dangerous physical diseases transfer into

insanity. The mental symptoms develop rapidly and often degenerate into melancholy or raving madness, while the threatening bodily symptoms vanish or diminish to such an extent that they seem to be replaced by perfect health (except to a gifted and persevering observer). They are like local one-sided diseases where the mental symptoms become the main symptom substituting and palliating the physical.

217. In these diseases examine all phenomena carefully, both the bodily symptoms and the precise character of the chief symptom of the mind and disposition. Select a remedy similar to the physical and to the mental and emotional state.

218. Obtain an accurate description of all the physical symptoms that existed before the disease degenerated into a one-sided mental disorder. This may come from the attendants of the patient.

219. Compare these previous symptoms with their remaining traces. They are now less perceptible but sometimes prominent when a lucid interval occurs, temporarily alleviating the mental picture. They are still present, but obscured.

220. By adding to this the state of mind and disposition we have completed the picture of the disease. We can now find a greatly similar remedy especially as regards the mental disturbance. If the mental disease has lasted a long time we must look among the antipsoric remedies.

221. If insanity has suddenly broken out as an acute disease, (sometimes caused by fright, vexation, drinking spirits, etc.) the patient normally being quite calm, do not at first treat with antipsorics even though it almost always arises from internal psora. Another class of remedies (*e.g.,* Aconite, Belladonna, Stramonium, Hyoscyamus, Mercury etc.) in high potency should be administered. These will

subdue it so far that the psora is for the present returned to its latent condition, so the patient will have appeared to have recovered.

222. Although relieved, they are not entirely cured by these non-antipsoric medicines. Do not lose any time[123] in perfecting the cure by continued antipsoric treatment, freeing the patient from the psoric miasm, which though latent is apt to break out anew. After treatment it will not break out again provided good diet and habits are followed.

> F/N 123: Rarely do long-term mental and emotional diseases cease spontaneously as the internal disease transfers itself to the physical organs. This is the case when a mental patient is discharged as cured. However *no-one is really permanently cured in an insane asylum*. Often homœopathy is able to restore mental and bodily health and return these patients to the world.

223. But if antipsoric treatment is omitted we can expect new, longer and more serious attacks of insanity resulting from much slighter causes. Psora usually then develops completely and may assume the form either of a periodical or continuous affection of the mind, which is then more difficult to cure with antipsorics.

224. When mental disease is not quite developed it is unclear whether it was caused by 1) a physical disease or 2) educational errors, bad habits, corrupt morals, neglected mental training, superstition or ignorance. If based on 2) it will yield to admonition, consolation, remonstrances and arguments. If caused by 1) they will be aggravated by admonition and become more exasperated.[124]

> F/N 124: It seems as if the mind feels uneasiness at the truth of these rational arguments and acts upon the body as if to restore lost harmony, but the body, by means of its disease, reacts upon the mind and puts them in greater disorder.

Emotional Disorders

225. There are however, some emotional disorders not developed from the physical but that originate and are sustained by emotional causes such as continual anxiety, worry, vexation, wrongs and the frequent occurrence of great fear and fright. This kind of disease will destroy physical health in time.

226. These, when they are *recent and have not undermined physical health* will allow a speedy cure by psychical remedies; such as a display of confidence, friendly exhortation, sensible advice and skilful deception; and with a healthy diet and regimen into a healthy state of body as well.

227. But these diseases are also founded upon the psoric miasm, not quite fully developed. For security's sake, subject the convalescent patient to thorough antipsoric treatment, to prevent re-occurrence.

228. In mental and emotional diseases resulting from physical diseases, which can only be cured by appropriate antipsoric treatment and a regulated mode of life, scrupulous behavior must be observed by those people around the patient. Meet furious mania with calm fearlessness and firmness of will; plaintive lamentation with silent commiseration in looks and gesture; senseless loquacity listen to in silence with some degree of attention; indecent behaviour and language by total inattention. Prevent destruction by removing articles *without reproaching the patient* and avoid all corporal punishment.[125] The homœopathic medicine can be administered by mixing it with the patient's usual drink if this is necessary.

F/N 125: A lament on the pitiful level of treatment in insane asylums.

229. Always treat mental patients *as if they are rational beings.*

Contradiction, explanations, rude correction, invective and timid yielding are all out of place. Nothing aggravates them more than force, argument or contempt and deception they can detect. Avoid all disturbance of the senses and mind. Nothing can soothe their troubled spirit, no wholesome distractions, instruction, conversation or books, except a cure, restoring them to health.[126]

> F/N 126: The treatment of the violently insane can only take place in an institution and not in the family.

230. If the antipsoric remedy selected for each case is quite homœopathic then a striking improvement will occur in no very long time. Indeed from experience, homœopathy can be demonstrated nowhere better than in mental and emotional diseases of long standing which came from physical diseases or were developed simultaneously with them.

Intermittent Diseases

231. *Intermittent diseases* also claim special attention as well as those that recur at definite periods (like the many kinds of intermittent fevers, and the apparently non-febrile affections that recur at intervals like intermittent fevers). Also there are morbid states which alternate with different morbid states at indefinite periods.

232. These latter, *alternating* diseases are also very numerous,[127] but all belong to the class of chronic diseases. They are generally a manifestation of developed psora, sometimes complicated with a syphilitic miasm. They can therefore usually be cured by antipsoric medicines, and in the latter case by sometimes alternating antipsorics with antisyphilitics. (see *Chronic Diseases*)

> F/N 127: (There follows a detailed description with examples, of different alternating disease situations). Two or three states may alternate with one another. When a state changes there is

often no trace of the previous state, or only a slight trace. Sometimes states are quite opposite in nature.

233. *Typical intermittent diseases* occur when a morbid state of unvarying character returns and departs at tolerably fixed periods, interspersed with apparent good health. This can be seen in apparently non-febrile morbid affections as well as intermittent fevers (febrile states).

234. These apparently non-febrile affections occurring in one patient at a time, do not appear sporadically or epidemically, but are always chronic and mostly psoric (they are rarely complicated with syphilis) and can be successfully treated as such when appearing in one patient at a time. Sometimes an intercurrent dose of potentised China is necessary to extinguish their intermittent nature.

235. In *intermittent fevers*[128] that prevail sporadically or epidemically (not those endemically located in marshy districts) we often see paroxysms of two opposite alternating states (cold, heat – heat, cold), or more often three stages (cold, heat, sweat). Therefore the remedy chosen (usually non-antipsoric) should be able to produce these successive stages and correspond with the most prominent and peculiar stage of the disease, either to the cold stage or to the hot or to the sweating stage and its accessory symptoms. But the patient's symptoms in the intervals, when the patient is free of fever must be the chief guide to the most appropriate remedy.[129]

> F/N 128: A description of the many various fevers and the tendency for them all to be treated as one disease, often with Cinchona which through overdosing will produce its own disease.

> F/N 129: See Boenninghausen's *An Attempt at Homœopathic Therapeutics of Intermittent Fevers*, 1833.

236. In these cases the medicine is best administered after the end of the paroxysms when the patient has partially recovered from it. The remedy will have time to work quietly during the intermission. If given before the next paroxysm it would coincide with the renewal of the disease and create distress to the point of possibly endangering life.[130]

> F/N 130: Illustrated in cases where small doses of Opium given during the cold stage have speedily killed the patient.

237. If the interval is very short as in some very bad fevers, or disturbed by the effects of the previous paroxysm, the remedy should be given when the perspiration begins to diminish or when the subsequent effects of the paroxysm begin to diminish.

238. One dose may destroy several attacks and restore health but more frequently another dose must be administered after each attack. Better still, when the character of the symptoms has not changed, doses of the same medicine may be given according to the newer discovery of repetition of doses (see note to § 270). Each successive dose is dynamised with 10-12 successions. There will sometimes (though seldom) be cases where the intermittent fever returns after several days well-being. This return of the same fever after a healthy interval is only possible when the noxious principle that first caused the fever is still acting upon the patient as is the case in marshy regions. Permanent restoration can only take place by moving away from the causative factor, by seeking a mountainous retreat (for instance).

239. Almost every medicine causes a peculiar type of fever different from the fever of other medicines (even intermittent fever with its alternating states). Medicines for a great many fevers exist even among the moderate amount of medicines already proved.

240. But if the remedy specific to an epidemic of intermittent fever does not perfectly cure and there is not a noxious marshy district

preventing the cure then it must be the psoric miasm in the background and antipsorics must be used to find complete relief.

241. Intermittent fever epidemics in places where none are endemic are chronic diseases composed of individual acute paroxysms. Each epidemic is of a uniform character common to all the individuals attacked, and when that character is found, the totality of symptoms indicate the specific remedy common to almost all the patients who enjoyed tolerable health before the epidemic; or at least those who were not chronic sufferers from developed psora.

242. If, in an epidemic, the first paroxysms of an intermittent fever have been uncured or weakened by allopathic treatment then the inherent latent psora existing in so many develops, and takes on the form of that type of intermittent fever. The medicine that was suitable for the first paroxysms (rarely antipsoric) is no longer suitable. We now have a psoric intermittent fever and this will generally be cured by rarely repeated doses of Sulphur and Hepar Sulphuris in high potency.

243. In a pernicious intermittent fever attacking a single person not living in a marshy district, we must *at first,* as in the case of acute diseases generally, select a remedy from the non-antipsorics. If there is no recovery we know we are dealing with psora on the point of its development and we must therefore use antipsoric medicines.

244. Healthy, young people can remain healthy if their habits are temperate, even in marshy districts or districts where fevers often take place. Endemic intermittents will attack such persons only as newcomers, but one or two doses of potentised China will cure the fever provided the well-regulated mode of life is continued. If it does not then the case if based on psora and will be cured by antipsorics.[131] Sometimes if this type of patient moves to a healthy climate they will apparently recover as long as the disease is not too deeply seated, *i.e.,* the psora resumes its latent state if it was not completely developed in

them. But they will never regain perfect health without antipsoric treatment.

> F/N 131: Large, frequent doses of Cinchona bark, or other concentrated Cinchonic remedies, such as *Sulphate of Quinine,* will free patients from periodical fevers but they will not cure, as they remain diseased in another way, frequently with an incurable Quinine intoxication. (see note to § 276)

Applying and Repeating Curative Remedies – LM Potencies

245. We will now consider curative remedies, how to apply them and the regimen to be observed during their use.

246. Do not repeat a remedy as long as there is a progressive and strikingly increasing amelioration. This is not infrequently the case in acute diseases. In chronic diseases a single dose will sometimes complete the cure naturally within 40-100 days. This is rare, however, and both physician and patient would like to diminish this period if possible. This can be done under the following conditions:
a) the remedy is perfectly homœopathic;
b) the remedy is highly potentised, dissolved in water, and *the degree of each dose differs from the proceeding and following dose* so that a medicinal disease is not precipitated. As is the case with rapidly repeated doses of the same potency. [132]

> F/N 132: What I said in the fifth edition, in order to prevent undesirable reactions of the vital energy, was all the experience I then had. In the last five years those difficulties have been solved by my altered but perfected method. The same carefully selected medicine may now be given daily and for months. After the lower degree of potency has been used for one or two weeks, we can advance to higher degrees (beginning according to the new dynamisation method, taught herewith with the use of the lowest degrees).

247. It is impractical to repeat the same unchanged dose of a remedy, once or frequently. The first dose changes the vital force and the same medicine repeated will not find the same conditions existing. In fact the patient may become sick from medicinal symptoms. But if the following doses are potentised higher each time (§§ 269-270) then the vital force can be altered without difficulty by the same medicine and bring the cure nearer.[133]

> F/N 133: Do not give the correct remedy dry in the same potency. Do not give the correct remedy dissolved in water in repeated doses from a bottle that has been *standing undisturbed* - it would not be beneficial even though it had originally been potentised with ten succussions. *But through modifying every dose in its degree of dynamisation* there is no offense even if doses are repeated frequently and highly potentised by many succussions. It seems as if the best remedy cures best *if applied in several different forms.*

248. For this purpose we potentise anew the medicinal solution[134] (with perhaps 8, 10, or 12 succussions) from which we give the patient one or (increasingly) several teaspoon doses in:
a) long-lasting diseases: daily or every second day;
b) acute diseases: every two to six hours;
c) very urgent cases: every hour or oftener.
In chronic disease we can give the correct remedy daily for months with increasing success. When used up (in seven to fifteen days) dissolve several pellets of a higher potency and continue as long as there is improvement. If the patient begins to experience a complaint he has never had before in a group of *altered* symptoms, then *another more homœopathic medicine must be chosen and administered in the same repeated, increasingly potentised doses.* Should there appear toward the end of treatment an *aggravation* (§ 161) of the original symptoms, this will be due to the medicine and doses should be reduced in frequency or even stopped for a few days in order to see if the patient needs any

further medicine. These apparent symptoms will soon disappear leaving health in their wake. If administering the remedy by olfaction (a globule having been dissolved in a dram of alcohol) this must also be successed 8-10 times before each olfaction.

> F/N 134: Made in 40, 30, 20, 15 or 8 tablespoons of water with some alcohol or a piece of charcoal. When using charcoal, suspend it by thread in the vial. Take it out when the vial is successed. The solution of the medicinal globule (it is rarely necessary to use more than one) of a thoroughly potentised medicine in a large quantity of water can be avoided by making a solution in only 7-8 tablespoons of water and after *thorough succussion of the vial* take from it one tablespoon and put it in a glass of water (containing 7 to 8 spoonfuls), *stir thoroughly* and then give a dose to the patient. If he is unusually excited and sensitive, a teaspoonful of this solution may be put in a second glass of water, thoroughly stirred and teaspoonful doses or more be given. There are patients of so great sensitiveness that a third or fourth glass, similarly prepared, may be necessary. Each such prepared glass must be made fresh daily. The globule of the high potency is best crushed in a few grains of sugar of milk which the patient can put in the vial and be dissolved in the required quantity of water.

Aggravations

249. Medicines prescribed for a case which produce new and troublesome symptoms will not cure properly.[135] If a medicine causes a considerable aggravation it must be reduced by an antidote before giving the next remedy. If the aggravation is not very violent give the next remedy immediately.[136]

> F/N 135: As experience shows a remedy cannot be prepared too small to effect an amelioration of a disease (§§ 275-278), we would be wrong to repeat the remedy or follow the old school

practice of *increasing the dose,* when there is no improvement or a slight aggravation, under the delusion that it was too small a dose. *Every aggravation that produces new symptoms* (when nothing has changed in the physical and mental regimen) *invariably proves the unsuitability of the medicine given, but never indicates that the dose has been too weak.*

F/N 136: The well informed and conscientiously careful physician will never require an antidote if he gives the selected medicine in the smallest possible dose. The better chosen remedy will re-establish order throughout.

250. When it is evident in urgent cases after six, eight or twelve hours that the remedy has been a poor choice, and that the patient is becoming worse (however slightly) with new symptoms and sufferings, then we must select the most appropriate remedy possible for the existing state of the disease, not something merely tolerably suitable (see § 167).

No Reaction

251. Some medicines (*e.g.,* Ignatia, Bryonia, Rhus Toxicodendron and sometimes Belladonna) affect the health principally in alternating actions, primary-action symptoms that are in part opposed to each other. If, after prescribing a dose of one of these, there is no improvement and you are sure of the strict homœopathicity of the remedy, repeat the same dose (in acute diseases after a few hours).[137]

F/N 137: As I have detailed more fully in the introduction to 'Ignatia', first volume *Materia Medica Pura.*

252. But if, when using the other medicines in chronic psoric diseases, the correct (antipsoric) remedy does not react it is a *sure* indication that the cause that keeps up the disease still persists – some circumstance in the patient's life or situation which must be removed

before a permanent cure can occur.

Signs of Improvement or Aggravation

253. The condition of the mind and general behaviour of the patient is the most certain sign of improvement or aggravation in all diseases, especially acute diseases. Increased comfort, tranquillity and freedom of mind, high spirits and a return to the natural state indicates improvement; a constrained, helpless and pitiable state of the disposition, mind, demeanour, gestures, postures and actions, the opposite, an aggravation.[138]

> F/N 138: Large material doses of the homœopathic remedy will produce too great a disturbance to allow us to immediately notice an improvement to the mind and disposition . A *sufficiently minute* dose will produce a perceptible improvement in the mind and disposition soon after the medicine has been taken.

254. We can distinguish improvement from aggravation by the appearance of new symptoms, an increase of those already present, or on the contrary, by the diminution of original symptoms undisturbed by new ones, even though patients are sometimes incapable of noticing or confessing either.

255. Even with such patients we can satisfy ourselves by re-examining them on every symptom in the case. If no new symptoms have appeared and old ones have not worsened, and especially if the state of mind and disposition has improved, the remedy has begun to work or soon will. But if improvement has been delayed beyond expectation, and one is sure of the remedy, then there is some fault in the regimen of the patient, or other interfering circumstances.

256. If, on the other hand, new and important symptoms occur, then the remedy is not homœopathic even though the patient may assure us

he is feeling better. As is the case, sometimes, in phthisical patients with lung abscess. We must regard their state as aggravated.

Treatment – General Advice

257. Avoid using 'favourite' remedies because they have often, by chance, been successful. We neglect other medicines which although less frequently used are often more homœopathic.

258. Do not reject remedies because they have not worked in particular cases. The fault is yours by not selecting them correctly. The only correct remedy is the one most similar to the characteristic symptoms of the case.

259. The minuteness of a remedy necessitates that every other medicinal influence in the *diet and regimen* must be avoided so that the dose is not counteracted.[139]

> F/N 139: The softest tones of a distant flute that in the still midnight hours would inspire a tender heart with exalted feelings and dissolve it in religious ecstasy, are inaudible and powerless amid discordant cries and the noise of the day.

260. Therefore in chronic cases especially look for noxious influences and other disease-causing errors in the diet and regimen which usually aggravate their diseases. They often pass unnoticed.[140]

> F/N 140: (A comprehensive list of substances and influences likely to disrupt or antidote a remedy and as far as possible to be removed or avoided). Some of my disciples increase the patient's dietry difficulties by forbidding the use of many more, tolerably indifferent, things. This is not commended.

261. During the treatment of chronic diseases, remove all obstacles to recovery and substitute a wholesome mode of life, innocent moral and

intellectual recreations, active exercise in the open air in almost all weathers (daily walks, slight manual labour), and suitable, nutritious food and drink unadulterated with medicines.

262. In acute diseases on the other hand, except in cases of mental alienation, the instinct of the patient should be followed. Gratify the patient's desires for food, without trying to persuade him to have anything injurious. The awakened life preserving principle knows what it needs.

263. In acute diseases, the patient's desire for food and drink is generally for things which palliate, they are not medicinal but gratify a sort of want. Any obstacles which they may place in the way of recovery[141] *within moderate bounds* is more than counterbalanced by the remedy's effects and the refreshment of taking what is longed for. Room temperature and coverings should be according to the patient's wishes, but avoid any mental over-exertion or emotional excitement.

> F/N 141: This is, however, rare; for instance, in pure inflammatory diseases, where Aconite is so indispensable, whose action would be antidoted by eating vegetable acids, the patient usually only wants cold water.

How to Prepare Genuine Remedies

264. We should have only *genuine remedies of unimpaired strength* so we can rely upon their therapeutic powers. We must *ourselves* be able to judge their genuineness.

265. We must ensure that the patient takes the correct remedy by preparing it and giving it to the patient ourselves.

266. Substances from the animal and vegetable kingdom possess their medicinal qualities most perfectly in their raw state.[142]

F/N 142: (A detailed description of how various animal and vegetable substances lose their varying medicinal properties during their preparation as food).

267. The active principles of freshly gathered plants are perfectly obtained by mixing their expressed juice *immediately* with equal parts of spirits of wine (95 degree grain alcohol). Wait 24 hours until the deposits have settled in a stopped bottle and decant off the clear fluid.[143] The alcohol will stop further fermentation of the vegetable juice preserving all medicinal power *for ever* in well corked bottles protected with wax and kept out of the sunlight.[144]

F/N 143: Alcohol has been used for making extracts to preserve vegetable juices for some time, but never as a way of administering them. (Hahnemann is referring to the fact that he was the first to do this).

F/N 144: Equal parts of alcohol and fresh juice are usually the best proportions for making the fibrous and albuminous matter deposit. But for plants that contain a lot of thick mucus *(e.g., Symphytum, Viola Tricolor)* or albumin *(e.g., Aethusa Cynapium, Solanum Nigrum)* a double proportion of alcohol is generally necessary. Plants that are deficient in juice *(Oleander, Buxus, Taxus, Ledum, Sabina)* must first be pounded up into a moist fine mass and then stirred up with a double quantity of alcohol, so that the juice combines with it, and being extracted by the alcohol, may be pressed out; these may also, when dried, be brought with milk-sugar to the millionfold trituration and then be further diluted and potentised (§ 271).

268. Don't use powdered barks, seeds and roots of foreign plants which cannot be obtained freshly without assuring yourself of their genuineness. Do this by examining them in their crude and complete state before using them medicinally.[145]

F/N 145: Well-dried animal and vegetable substances still contain a certain amount of moisture and will spoil even in well-corked bottles. When the powdered substance is finely pulverised a somewhat moist powder will appear which must be separated. Do this by spreading out the powder in a flat tin saucer with a raised edge, which floats in a vessel full of boiling water (*i.e.,* a water bath), and by means of stirring it about, drying it to such a degree that all the small atoms of it no longer stick together in lumps but like dry, fine sand are easily separated from each other and are readily converted into dust. In this dry state the powders can be kept *forever* in well-corked and sealed bottles, retaining their medicinal power *without being injured by mites or mould.* Keep the bottles away from daylight in covered boxes, chests or cases. If you do not keep them away from sunlight or air-tight they will gradually lose their medicinal power.

269. The homœopathic system develops the inner medicinal powers of crude substances by a process which has never before been tried, whereby they become remedial[146] *even when in their crude state there is no evidence of the slightest medicinal power.* These slumbering,[147] hidden, dynamic (§ 11) powers influence the life principle and change the well-being of animal life.[148] This occurs through the mechanical action on their smallest particles by rubbing (trituration) and shaking (succussion) *and through the addition of an indifferent substance, dry or fluid.* This process is called dynamising, potentising (development of medicinal power) and the products are dynamisations[149] or potencies in different degrees.

F/N 146: The change in substances by friction has long been known, *e.g.,* warmth, heat, fire, development of odour in odourless objects, magnetism of steel, etc. But these relate only to physical, inanimate things. There is a law of nature whereby physiological and pathogenic changes can be caused in the body by forces generated in the crude material of drugs through succussion and trituration, even drugs that have never shown any medicinal properties. This is conditional upon their being dissolved in a non-medicinal vehicle in fixed proportions.

F/N 147: The same thing is seen in a bar of iron and steel where a trace of a latent magnetic force cannot be recognised. To *dynamise* it fully one has to rub it with a dull file *in one direction*. In the same way trituration and succussion develop the hidden medicinal powers of a substance. One could say that the process spiritualises the material substance.

F/N 148: This can only happen if the body comes into contact with the remedy by intake or olfaction. Just like the magnetic power of the iron bar is only perceptible when a steel needle is near enough to be attracted to it. Dynamised medicines have no effect on *lifeless things* as the magnet has no effect on brass.

F/N 149: Homœopathic remedies are not *mere dilutions*. They are a true opening up of the substances, revealing their hidden specific medicinal powers by rubbing and shaking. The non-medical dilutant is only a *secondary* though indispensable factor. Mere dilution without dynamisation will not produce medicinal substances.

270. In order to best dynamise a substance, a small part, say one grain (0.064798918 grams Troy or 0.062 Nuremburg measure) is triturated for three hours with three times one hundred grains of sugar of milk according to the method described below[150] to the one-millionth part in powder form. For reasons given below one grain of this powder is dissolved in 500 drops of a mixture of one part of alcohol (brandywine equivalent to 90 degree grain alcohol) and four parts of distilled water, and *one drop* of that is put into a vial. To this are added 100 drops of pure alcohol[151] (rectified wine spirit equivalent to 95 degree grain

alcohol), and given 100 strong succussions with the hand against a hard but elastic body.[152] This produces the *first* degree of dynamisation with which small sugar globules[153] may then be moistened,[154] quickly spread on blotting paper to dry and kept in well-corked vials labelled (I) degree of potency. Only one[155] globule of this is taken for further dynamisation, put in a second new vial (with a drop of water to dissolve it) and then with 100 drops of 95 degree alcohol and dynamised in the same way with 100 powerful succussions, then label (II) or second degree of potency. The process is repeated in the same way until the 30th is reached. By means of this procedure even unmedicinal materials can be changed into spirit-like[156] medicines, *not perceptible* to our senses. The dry medicated globule acts as *the carrier* and manifests the healing power of this invisible force in the sick body. This is manifested even more so when dissolved in water.

F/N 150: One third of one hundred grains of sugar of milk is put in a glazed porcelain mortar, the bottom previously dulled by rubbing with a fine, moist sand. *Upon this powder* is put one grain of the powdered drug to be triturated (Quicksilver, Petroleum, etc.). The sugar of milk must be of a special pure quality, crystallised on strings. To begin with mix the medicine and powder with a porcelain spatula, then triturate strongly for six to seven minutes with a porcelain pestle, roughened dull. Then the mass is scraped from the bottom of the mortar and the pestle for three or four minutes in order to make it homogeneous. Follow by triturating in the same way for another 6-7 minutes and again scraping for 3-4 minutes the mortar and pestle. Add the second third of the sugar of milk, mixed with the spatula, triturated for 6-7 minutes, scraped for 3-4 minutes and again triturated for 6-7 minutes. Add the last third of sugar of milk, mix with the spatula, and triturate for 6-7 minutes carefully scraping the mixture together. The resulting powder is put in a vial, corked well, protected from the light and marked 1/100 (IC). To raise this to 1/10,000

(IIC), one grain of the 1/100 is mixed with 1/3 of 100 grains of milk of sugar and one proceeds as before. Ensure each third is triturated strongly twice, for 6/7 minutes before the next third is added followed by 3-4 minutes of scraping. When finished we have 1/1,000,000 (IIIC), each grain containing 1/1,000,000 of the original substance. This trituration to the third degree required 6 times 6-7 minutes for trituration, and 6 times 3-4 minutes for scraping, or one hour for each degree. Mortar, pestle and spatula must be cleaned thoroughly before being used for another medicine. Wash first with warm water and dry. Then put in boiling water for half and hour. To be sure one might even put the utensils in a coal fire and expose to glowing heat.

F/N 151: The vial used for potentising is filled two thirds full.

F/N 152: Perhaps a leather bound book.

F/N 153: The globules are prepared from starch and sugar and freed from fine dusty parts by passing them through a sieve. Then put them through a strainer that allows only 100 to pass through weighing one grain.

F/N 154: A small cylindrical vessel shaped like a thimble, made of glass, porcelain or silver, with a small opening at the bottom in which the globules to be medicated are put. They are moistened with some of the dynamised medicinal alcohol, stirred and poured out on blotting paper, in order to dry them quickly.

F/N 155: According to my first directions, one drop of the liquid of a lower potency was to be taken to 100 drops of 95 degree alcohol for higher potentisation. However this proportion was found too limited to develop thoroughly to a high degree without using great force in succussion. If one takes only one, one grain globule and dynamises it with 100 drops of 95 degree alcohol, then the proportion becomes 1/50,000, or even higher, because 500, one grain globules hardly absorb one drop. With this higher ratio many succussive strokes can produce a much greater development of power. Medicines produced at a ratio of 100:1 act almost immediately with furious or even dangerous violence, especially in weaker patients, without having a lasting mild reaction of the vital force. The 50,000:1 method produces powerful medicines of the mildest action, touching all suffering parts curatively. Although, in rare cases, notwithstanding almost full recovery and good vital strength, an old local trouble may continue. In such a case it is necessary to administer the remedy, already proved efficacious, in increasingly larger doses potentised to a very high degree by means of *many* succussions by hand. The local disease will often then disappear. In acute fevers, the small doses of the lowest dynamisation of these medicines, even of long continued action (like Belladonna), may be repeated at short intervals. In chronic diseases it is best to begin with the lowest degrees of dynamisation and when necessary advance to higher.

F/N 156: Not improbable if one considers that the material part of the medicine is lessened with each degree of dynamisation 50,000 times and yet increases in power, so that the further dynamisation of 125×10^{18} reaches only the third degree of dynamisation. The thirtieth therefore gives a fraction almost impossible to express in numbers. The material part dissolves into its spirit-like essence, which was undeveloped in its crude state.

271. If the practitioner prepares the medicines himself, as he should,[157] he can use the fresh plant, as only a small amount of the

crude substance is needed, unless we happen to need the extracted juice for treatment. Take a few grains of the fresh plant in a mortar with 100 grains of sugar of milk and three distinct times bring them to the millionth trituration (§ 270) before further potentisation with a small portion by shaking (succussion), a procedure to also be observed with all medicinal substances of a dry or oily nature.

F/N 157: Until the State, in the future, has homœopathic medicines prepared perfectly and gives them to homœopathic physicicans trained in homœopathic hospitals, their being examined theoretically and practically and legally qualified. Physicians may then be convinced of these divine healing tools and give them free of charge to their patients – rich and poor.

The Single Dose

272. Such a globule,[158] placed dry upon the tongue is one of the smallest doses for a moderate recent case of illness. But only a few nerves are touched by the medicine. A globule, crushed with some sugar of milk and dissolved in a good deal of water (§ 247) and stirred well before every administration will produce a far more powerful medicine for use over several days. Every dose will touch many nerves.

F/N 158: These globules (§ 270) retain their medicinal value for *many* years if protected against sunlight and heat.

273. It is *not permissable* to administer more than one *single, simple*[159] *medicine* at one time. Never mix several differently acting drugs.

F/N 159: This rule excludes neutral and intermediate salts formed through chemical affinity from two opposite substances in unchanged proportions (sulphuretted metals and compounds of sulphur with alkaline salts), those produced artificially by combining Sulphur and alkaline salts and earths (Natrum

Sulphuricum and Calcarea Sulphuricum), and ethers produced by distillation of alcohol and acids together with Phosphorus. Consider them as simple medicinal substances and use them for patients. However, so called alkaloids of plants extracted with acids are exposed to great variety in their preparation (Quinine, Strychnine, Morphine) and cannot be accepted as *simple* medicines, always the same, especially as we already have them in plants in their natural state (Peruvian bark, Nux Vomica, Opium). Alkaloids are not the only constituents of plants.

274. It is useless to apply a multiplicity where simplicity will suffice. By mixing drugs it is impossible to foresee the variety of possible effects they may produce. Simple single medicines will give relief, their totality of symptoms being *thoroughly proved*. Even a poorly selected remedy can sometimes call forth new symptoms in a case, corroborating provings on that remedy – something you cannot see with compounds.[160]

F/N 160: And if the correct remedy is given it is irrational to have the patient drink infusions of different plants, inject medicated enemas or rub in this or that ointment.

275. The appropriateness of a remedy not only depends upon its homœopathicity but also its proper size or smallness of the dose. *Too strong a dose,* though homœopathic, will produce an injurious effect on the vital force which in turn acts upon those sensitive parts of the organism most affected by the disease.

276. It will be injurious not only due to the large dose but also due to the degree of potentisation[161] of the medicine. It will be more harmful than an unsuitable unhomœopathic, allopathic medicine unrelated to the disease. Too large doses of the correct remedy, especially when frequently repeated, bring about much trouble as a rule. They endanger the patient or make his disease incurable. They extinguish

the natural disease but replace it with the similar but more violent medicinal *disease which* is more difficult to destroy.[162]

> F/N 161: The praise bestowed by some homœopaths on the larger doses is either because they chose low dynamisations of the medicine (as I used to do 20 years ago, knowing no better) or that the medicine was not homœopathic and imperfectly prepared by the manufacturers.

> F/N 162: Continuous large, allopathic doses of Mercury given against syphilis develop almost incurable mercurial diseases, when one or several doses of a mild but active mercurial preparation would have cured the whole venereal disease in a few days, provided the chancre had not been destroyed by external measures. Similarly the allopath gives Peruvian bark and Quinine in intermittent fever daily in large doses where correctly indicated, but where one small dose of highly potentised China would have unfailingly helped (in marsh intermittents and even in patients not affected by any evident psoric disease). Instead a chronic China disease coupled with the development of psora is produced which, if it does not kill the patient by damaging important internal organs, will cause years of ill health. An homœopathic antidote for this abuse of large doses of homœopathic remedies is hardly conceivable.

277. For the same reason the closely homœopathic remedy will better cure the more its dose is reduced to the appropriate degree of minuteness for a gentle remedial effect.

278. Which begs the question as to how much must a medicine be reduced? Only pure experiment, careful observation of the sensitivity of each patient and accurate experience *in each individual case,* can answer this.

279. If there is no considerable deterioration to a vital organ, and if all other alien medicines are kept from the patient, the dose can never be made so small that it is not stronger than, and cannot overpower a disease at least partly, and so begin a cure; even in chronic and complicated diseases.

Repetition of the Dose

280. The remedy should be continued in *gradually ascending* doses (§ 247) as long as the patient *improves generally*, with no new troublesome symptoms, and begins to feel mildly the return of one or more old original complaints. This indicates an approaching cure. The vital force no longer needs to be affected by the similar medicinal disease in order to lose the sensation of the natural disease (§ 148). The vital force now free from the natural disease, only suffers from the medicinal disease, *i.e.,* the *homœopathic aggravation.*

281. In order to verify this, leave the patient without medicine for eight, ten or fifteen days, giving him some powders of sugar of milk while continuing good hygienic regulations. If the complaints are due to the medicine stimulating the original disease symptoms, they will disappear in a few days or hours and he is probably cured. If traces of the original disease return, continue with higher potencies of the remedy. Again gradually raise the potencies, less so and more slowly in patients where considerable irritability is evident than in those of less susceptibility, where we can advance to higher potencies more quickly. There are patients whose impressionability compared to that of the unsusceptible is of the ratio 1,000 to 1.

282. It is a definite sign that the dose is too large, especially in chronic diseases, if a so called *homœopathic aggravation* (an increase of the original symptoms) occurs after every dose (§ 247), even though each dose was modified by succussion before administration.[163]

F/N 163: The rule to begin treatment of chronic diseases with the smallest possible doses and to gradually increase their strength does not apply to the treatment of the three great miasms while they still manifest on the skin, *i.e., itch* (scabies), *chancre* (on the sexual organs, labia, mouth or lips etc.) and *fig-warts.* These will only tolerate, and indeed require from the beginning, large doses of their specific remedies in higher and higher potencies daily or several times a day. If this is done there is no danger of producing a chronic medicinal disease. The daily progress of the treatment can be observed and we can judge the progress of the cure as the disease disappears. None of these three can be cured without convincing the physician, by the disappearance of their external manifestations, that there is no longer any need for medicine. Diseases in general, are a dynamic attack upon the life principle and nothing material. There is nothing material to be taken away without making the patient more incurable *(Chronic Diseases Part 1).* This dynamic attack is the essence of the external signs of an illness and can be extinguished solely by homœopathic medicines, curing the patient. Experience teaches us that the itch (scabies) and chancre can only be cured by internal medicines, but figwarts, if they have existed for some time without treatment, will need external applications of their specific medicines at the same time as internal use for a perfect cure.

283. In order to work according to nature only prescribe remedies in the smallest doses. If we give the wrong remedy the effect will be so small that the patient will be able to repair any bad effects through his own vital powers and our early prescription (§ 249) of the correct remedy.

How to Administer the Remedy

284. The tongue, mouth and stomach are most commonly affected by taking a remedy. The nose and respiratory organs are receptive to

remedies in a fluid form taken by olfaction and inhalation through the mouth. The skin and epidermis of the whole body is also sensitive to remedies especially if rubbed in simultaneously with internal administration.[164]

> F/N 164: Medicines work very well on babies through the milk of the mother or wet nurse. Every disease of the baby will be cured by administering remedies to the nursing mother much more easily than in later years. Psora is given to babies through the milk of the nurse if not already inherited from the mother, and can be cured in the same manner. But if mothers are treated in their first pregnancy with mild antipsorics (especially Sulphur potencies prepared according to § 270) then both mother and fœtus will be cured, and healthier and stronger children will be born.

285. We can cure very old diseases more rapidly by rubbing the remedy into the back, arms, and extremities as well as taking it internally. But avoid doing so to parts affected by pain, eruptions or spasms.[165]

> F/N 165: This explains cures on chronic deformed patients in mineral baths (spas) by chance, through their containing homœopathically related constituents. On the other hand they *very often* bring increased injury through suppressing eruptions. After brief improvement the uncured malady appears somewhere else in more important organs. Sometimes the ocular nerve paralyses producing blindness for no apparent reason, or the lens becomes cloudy, hearing loss, mania or suffocating asthma follows, or apoplexy kills the patient. Homœopaths never use anything on a patient that has not been proved (§§ 20 & 21). We must therefore *never* send patients to mineral baths because we do not know their full effects.

Magnetism

286. Magnets, electricity and galvanism act as powerfully on the vital force and are no less homœopathic than remedies taken orally, through olfaction or by rubbing into the skin. There may be diseases such as those of sensibility and irritability, abnormal sensations, and involuntary muscular movements which can be cured by these means. But at the moment we know too little of the homœopathic effects upon the healthy of electricity, galvanism and the electro-magnetic machine for us to make use of them.

287. We can more reliably use magnets as detailed in *Materia Medica Pura,* by the positive effects of the north and south poles of a powerful magnetic bar. Both poles are equally powerful but they oppose each other in the their effects. We can modify the dosage by the length of time in contact with one or the other pole, according to which pole's symptoms are indicated. If it is necessary to antidote, apply a plate of polished zinc.

Mesmerism

288. *Animal magnetism* or *Mesmerism* acts in a quite different way from all the other therapeutic agents. The strong will of a well-intentioned mermerist by contact, or at some distance, can bring healthy energy into the patient dynamically (just like one of the poles of a magnet on a bar of steel). It works partly by replacing deficient energy, or pushing aside and diminishing the over-accumulation of vital force in some parts that produced irritating, nervous disorders. It distributes the vital force equally and generally extinguishes the morbid condition, substituting it with the normal condition of the hypnotist, *e.g.,* in conditions such as old ulcers, blindness with no known cause, paralysis of single organs, etc. This has been shown most brilliantly by the resuscitation of people who have lain apparently dead for some time, by the powerful will of a man full of vital energy.[166] A good-natured mesmerist can at times perform apparent miracles.

F/N 166: Especially in people who are kind, have perfect bodily powers and possess only *a very moderate desire for sexual intercourse.* Consequently a great deal of energy can be directed to others by touch and powerful exertion of the will. *All* the powerful mesmerisers I have met had these characteristics.

289. The above methods depend on an influx of vital energy into the patient and are therefore called positive mesmerism.[167] There is the opposite effect, negative mesmerism. The passes used to wake a sleepwalker as well as the hand movements known as *soothing and ventilating* belong to this class. This *discharge* is made by making a very rapid motion of the flat extended hand, held parallel to, and about an inch distant from the body, from the top of the head to the tips of the toes.[168] The more rapid the pass, the more effective the discharge. In a case of a previously healthy[169] woman with suppressed periods caused by a violent mental shock, who lay apparently dead, the vital force, probably accumulated in the precordial region, was discharged and equilibrium restored by rapid negative passes; the patient resuscitated immediately.[170] In the same way a gentle, less rapid, negative pass reduces the excessive restlessness, sleeplessness and anxiety sometimes produced in very irritable people by a too powerful positive pass.

F/N 167: I do not mean the deplorable application of it where passes are made for half an hour or an hour at a time, day after day, which induces in weak nervous people a somnambulant state which loosens them from normal sensitivity and seems to belong to the world of spirits – an unnatural and dangerous state, by means of which attempts are made to cure chronic diseases.

F/N 168: A subject to be mesmerised, positively or negatively, should not wear silk on any part of the body.

F/N 169: A negative pass, especially if very rapid, is very

injurious to a delicate person affected with a chronic ailment and deficient in vital force.

F/N 170: A ten year old, strong country boy because of a slight indisposition, received several very powerful passes with the points of both thumbs from a female mesmerist, from the pit of the stomach along the lower edge of the ribs. He instantly grew very pale and fell deeply unconscious, and was given up for dead. I made his elder brother give him a very rapid negative pass from the crown of his head over the body to the feet, and he immediately recovered and became lively and well.

Massage

290. Massage by a healthy good-natured person on a chronic invalid, cured but still suffering from loss of flesh, weak digestion and lack of sleep, due to slow convalescence, is also a mesmeric influence and should not be used to excess in still hypersensitive patients. The muscles of the limbs, breast and back, separately grasped and moderately pressed and kneaded arouses the life principle and reaches and restores the tone of the muscles and blood and lymph vessels.

Baths

291. Baths of pure water are partly palliative and aid in restoring health in acute disease and convalescence of cured chronic cases. Be careful with the condition of the convalescent and the temperature of the bath, its duration and repetition. In themselves they are not a medicine but bring physical beneficial changes. Lukewarm baths of 25-27 R. (Réaumur) (31-34 degrees Centigrade) resuscitate the apparently dead (the frozen, drowned or suffocated). Although only palliative, they often prove active, especially when given at the same time as coffee and rubbing with the hands. They may give homœopathic aid in cases where the irritability is very unevenly distributed and accumulated unevenly in some organs as is the case in

some hysteric spasms, and infantile convulsions. Similarly taking cold *instantaneous* baths of 10 to 6 R. (13-7 degrees Centigrade) in cured chronic patients deficient in vital heat, has acted as an homœopathic aid. Later they should take *repeated* baths for more than an instant - for some minutes - and at a gradually lowered temperatures. The baths act as a physical palliative restorative to the tone of the exhausted fibre, and have no connection with the disadvantage of a reversed action as can take place afterwards with dynamic medicinal palliatives.

INDEX